SLEEP

the
gentle tyrant

Wilse B. Webb

Prentice-Hall, Inc. A SPECTRUM BOOK   Englewood Cliffs, N.J.

Library of Congress Cataloging in Publication Data

WEBB, WILSE B
   Sleep, the gentle tyrant.

   (A Spectrum Book)
   Includes index.
   1. Sleep. I. Title.
QP425.W32   612'.821   75-25959
ISBN 0-13-812933-9
ISBN 0-13-812925-8 pbk.

PRENTICE-HALL INTERNATIONAL, INC. *(London)*
PRENTICE-HALL OF AUSTRALIA, PTY. LTD. *(Sydney)*
PRENTICE-HALL OF CANADA, LTD. *(Toronto)*
PRENTICE-HALL OF INDIA PRIVATE LIMITED *(New Delhi)*
PRENTICE-HALL OF JAPAN, INC. *(Tokyo)*
PRENTICE-HALL OF SOUTHEAST ASIA (PTE.) *(Singapore)*

1881104

Contents

5

The timing of sleep and waking

6

Conditions prior to and during sleep

7

Individual differences in sleep

8

The disorders of sleep

9

Sleep and pathological conditions

10

Drugs and sleep

11

The insomnias

Preface

It has been my good fortune to be in the midst of the exciting era of "Modern Sleep Research" that began in the late 1950s and early 1960s. This era has seen a great outpouring of research about sleep. Currently there are about 600 papers a year on the topic. However, as with any scientific assault on a complex phenomenon, much of this activity has been a clearing of underbrush, haring after false leads, enthusiastic championing of causes and, above all, has been piecemeal and highly technical. All of this has been necessary and natural. Unfortunately, as a consequence, the findings could be assessed only by experts and communicated only with difficulty. Most critically, in such affairs, the phenomenon itself tends to disappear in the same way that a pointillist painting disappears as each dot is examined. While examining each leaf or even each tree, the paths and the panorama of the forest are not seen.

However, I believe the time is approaching when we can begin to put together these complex details into a coherent picture in order to begin to understand the phenomenon of sleep and, in turn, use this information. That is what I have tried to do here.

There has been an ever-increasing stream of books about sleep in the last 10 years; there are some 25 on the table beside me right now. Most of them, however, are intergroup communications between the researchers—sort of grown-up "show and tell" sessions. There are a few general ones. I find fault with some of these because they are dated (sleep research has been fast-moving) and with others because they are too "textbookish" in their emphasis on particularized facts at the expense of the process and phenomenon of sleep.

What purpose do I want this book to serve? I want to tell people who have minimal technical expertise about the act of sleeping as it exists in their day-to-day lives and the variations in this behavior that they may be experiencing. I am concerned with the description of sleep, its variations, the factors that influence and determine it, and what difference it may make in our waking behavior.

A few notes of caution, reservation, and apology. The data of this book was selectively seined from well over 1,000 highly technical articles that I have read. Of course, the interpretations must be mine as well as the authors'. Moreover, even with these masses of data the answers to all the questions about sleep are by no means in or even yet asked. This makes for very real problems.

A research scientist who is trying to write a book for a more general readership than his fellow researchers is particularly plagued. In attempting to be clear he tries to avoid presumptions about research backgrounds, to reduce specialized terminologies, and to minimize complexities. In attempting to answer reasonable questions where research conclusions are less than certain or even lacking, he interjects his own judgments. He sails between the Scylla of superficiality and exaggeration and the Charybdis of cautionary overdetail. And humanly, he errs.

My apologies then: to the general reader for references to little-known, esoteric studies, for what may seem an excessive use of numbers, for background statements that I have found necessary; to my fellow sleep researchers for glossing over problems and speculations which extend beyond data. I have consciously tried to avoid gross offenses in either direction.

Will you sleep better after having read this book? I certainly think that it is possible. I believe sleep to be a beautiful part of our heritage as humans. It is a natural and I believe an increasingly understandable phenomenon. I would hope that a reading of this book would result in an understanding of the characteristics and rules of this great system. What you do with this understanding is, of course, up to you. I agree with Sir Francis Bacon, who said some 550 years ago: "Nature cannot be commanded except by being obeyed." Sleep on that.

Acknowledgments

There are desirable, necessary, and traditional acknowledgments to be made.

I certainly want to gratefully acknowledge the research support I have received that has made possible my learning about sleep over the last 15 years: the early support of the Air Force Office of Scientific Research, the long-term (but, alas, recently terminated) support of the National Institute of Mental Health, the vital and continued support of the National Aeronautics and Space Agency. The support of these and similar agencies has been the vital necessity for the creation of the sleep research by all of us that has made this book possible.

I continue to learn from my graduate students—in this era, Royce White, Mike Dube, and Mike Bonnett. Bob Agnew, my long-time collaborator, and Gail Clyne, our laboratory secretary, did much to order my self-created chaos. And my wife continues to contribute to my life in ways that permit me to be better than I really am.

Several publishers have kindly permitted the reprinting of excerpts or illustrations:

The quotation from *Sleep* by Gay Gaer Luce and Julius Segal is reprinted by permission of Coward McCann & Geoghegan, Inc., and William Heinemann. Copyright © 1966 by Gay Gaer Luce and Julius Segal.

The quotation from R. Pasnau et al., "The Psychological Effects of 205 Hours of Sleep Deprivation" is reprinted from the *Archives of*

General Psychiatry, April 1968, Volume 18, pp. 501–502 by permission of the publisher and the author. Copyright 1968, American Medical Association.

The quotation from *Experimental Studies of Dreaming*, H. Witkins and H. Lewis, editors, is reprinted by permission of Random House, Inc. Copyright © 1967 by Random House, Inc.

Six double-page illustrations and 59 lines of text from *Dr. Seuss's Sleep Book*, by Dr. Seuss, are reprinted by permission of Random House, Inc., and Collins Publishers. Copyright © 1962 by Dr. Seuss.

The illustration from *Chronobiology*, L. E. Scheving, J. E. Pauly, and F. Halberg, editors, is used by permission of Igaku Shoin Ltd.

1

Introduction and overview

There is no doubt that I am supersensitive to sleep. Like the politician who views the world in terms of votes, the botanist who sees flowers everywhere, or the mother who is constantly aware of her child, I am always hearing about sleep.

"I couldn't get to sleep last night."
"I slept through the alarm this morning."
"I stayed up for the late show."
"I'm on the late shift this week."
"I'm trying a new sleeping pill."
"The guy next door played his radio until two."
"Isn't nine hours of sleep every night too much?"
"My baby slept all night."
"I keep going to sleep in class."
"I had the craziest dream last night."
"How can a guy fly in from India and testify the next day?"
"I woke up feeling lousy this morning."
"I can't get Johnny to go to bed."
"Whenever I'm worried I can't sleep."
"I used to have no trouble sleeping."
"I wake up and can't get back to sleep."
"He wets his bed."
"I can't sleep in a motel."

Being identified with sleep through my work, I find the casual remarks extending to questions:

"I heard somebody stayed awake for ten days. Is it true?"
"Does studying all night for an exam hurt you at exam time?"
"My child has nightmares. What should I do?"

"How much sleep should I get?"

"Do bright people sleep less than dull ones?"

"I don't remember my dreams. Is something wrong?"

"I've started sleeping poorly. Can you recommend a sleeping pill?"

"Does this stuff that they advertise on television work?"

"What is sleepwalking?"

"I hear if you don't dream you go crazy."

"How can you tell if a person is asleep?"

Sometimes the questions get professional.

"What schedule do the astronauts sleep on?"

"What are the best shift-work schedules?"

"Is this drug any good?"

"How can we keep people on low-demand jobs awake?"

"Should day-care centers schedule one or two nap periods?"

"I am not sleeping well. Can you help me?"

Hardly a day goes by without my hearing about the pleasures or problems of sleeping.

Certainly there is good reason for this. Like the weather, like eating, like breathing, sleeping is a natural part of our existence. In fact, it occupies one-third of our lives.

However, because sleep is such a natural part of our day-to-day lives, coming and going like a well-trained servant, most of us forget its very large role in our lives. Unless we are among the unfortunates, the insomniacs whose servant has turned surly, we often ignore it. We should not. It is not only one of the most fascinating of our biological heritages, it is a sensitive and responsive system that is much abused in our time. Francis Bacon's description, in the 1500s, of our general physiology is most apt in describing sleep: "A musical instrument of much and exquisite workmanship easily put out of tune."

This book, to vary a popular phrase, is intended to tell you everything that you wanted to know about sleep and occasionally asked. I would hasten to add, however, that it does not tell you everything there is to know about sleep. The far-ranging research designed to illuminate this dark kingdom includes widely different concerns: the actions of single nerve cells in the brain, complex biochemical processes, central nervous system circuitry, the sleep of infants and the sleep of turtles, the use of drugs, the interpretation of dreams, and the sleep of shift workers, to name a few. While some of these will be considered here, we shall not include others. Basically we will be concerned with the role of sleep in our everyday lives.

This chapter presents the perspective of this book within the general context of sleep research and the phenomena of sleep to be covered.

Approaches to sleep

As with most of the natural and inherent aspects of living—in the absence of problems—our usual approach to sleep is to accept our endowment without thought or thanks. Like our water supply, our breathing, the weather, or our digestion, we pretty much take such things for granted. But occasionally we may do homage, as John Keats did in the early 1800s.

> To Sleep
> O soft embalmer of the still midnight,
> Shutting, with careful fingers and benign,
> Our gloom-pleas'd eyes, embower'd from the light,
> Enshaded in forgetfulness divine:
> O soothest Sleep! if so it please thee, close,
> In midst of this thine hymn, my willing eyes,
> Or wait the amen, ere thy poppy throws
> Around my bed its lulling charities.
> Then save me, or the passed day will shine
> Upon my pillow, breeding many woes;
> Save me from the curious conscience, that still lords
> Its strength for darkness, burrowing like a mole;
> Turn the key deftly in the oiled wards,
> And seal the hushed casket of my soul.

Oh, would it were always so! "Turn the key deftly in the oiled wards." Unfortunately, as the environmentalists have lately been impressing on us, nature may be disturbed. Furthermore, the many aspects of the modern world seem to lend themselves to disturbance— a fact perhaps easiest to note in regard to sleep. In what may seem an oversimplification, we go to sleep when we wish to but we wake up or stay awake when we must. The invention of the electric light, heralding the advent of the Edison Age, yielded fertile ground for extending our wishes well beyond the fall of darkness, and the invention of television added stimulation to that time. This has created an "around-the-clock" world, in which we may work at any time and must adjust our sleep accordingly. Jet aircraft toss us across multiple time zones and displace our sleep in turn. There are added noises, tensions, stimulations, drugs, and an extended aging process. No longer soothed by the gentle fingers of darkness, but rather surrounded by the cacophony of the times and tossed from time to time, it is small wonder that "gentle" sleep may be disturbed.

When faced with problems we try many solutions—prayer, politics, laws, common sense, education, and exhortation, to name a few. They often work; they sometimes don't. Since the early 1800s we have increasingly supplemented our efforts at solutions by the use of a powerful ally—science—or by the systematic gathering of data about our problems. Sleep research, though largely neglected until recently, has been a part of this enterprise.

The long, broad domain
of sleep research

As has been said of psychology, sleep research has a long memory but a short history. Until the late 1800s, sleep was largely the realm of poets and folklore. Even in its research beginnings, facts and theories about sleep were usually afterthoughts from new findings about human physiology. The later half of the nineteenth century and the early twentieth century saw rapid advances in physiology. From these new findings "new" theories of sleep would often emerge. They most frequently took their place under the "humoral-toxic" theories, or "inhibitory" theories. The first, emerging from new findings about the chemistry of man, invoked certain substances as a "trigger" or cause of sleep. In a 1963 review of the humoral-toxic theories, an author cited the presence of eighteen "substances" whose progressive buildup had been suggested as the cause of sleep. "Inhibitory" theories grew from our advances in understanding the central nervous system and posited changes in the central nervous system as the cause of sleep.

During this earlier period there was an overwhelming impression of sleep research as an orphan of uncertain parentage living within a larger family of powerful aunts and uncles who, occasionally, gave sustenance and attention to the waif.

The modern era of sleep research dates from the late 1950s. While scientific research in general was receiving unprecedented support, sleep research received extra impetus from a newly developed use of the electroencephalogram to "define" or measure sleep in both humans and animals and to measure dreams within sleep (Chapter 2).

The 1960s saw a veritable explosion of research on sleep. The number of scientific articles published about sleep before that time had been about 100 per year. This number has steadily increased each year until there are now about 600 articles annually. Between 1960 and 1965 there were 3 substantial books on sleep research published; in 1974 alone there were at least 8 such books.

Contemporary sleep research continues to be a stepchild of many disciplines but the central focus of none. Researchers drawn from a wide range of primary training and interests have been and are involved in the enterprise: biochemists, biologists, endocrinologists, neurologists, pediatricians, pharmacologists, physiologists, psychiatrists, psychologists, and engineers, to cite the more obvious.

The range, shifts in emphasis, and increase in effort can be seen in Table 1-1. This table displays the nature of the papers published about sleep from the 1920s to the present.

TABLE 1-1 Percentage Distribution of Sleep Publications in 4 Five-Year Periods by Areas of Research

	1926–1930	1946–1950	1962–1967	1968–1972
Brain neurology	10	14	24	17
Brain chemistry	13	15	13	20
General physiology	15	13	5	5
Sleep and pathology	26	19	14	16
Species and growth comparisons	10	7	7	8
Deprivation effects	3	1	13	9
Dream content	4	6	6	8
Miscellaneous*	20	26	16	17
Est. Number/Yr.	110	115	550	575

* General articles, instrumentation, electrosleep, hypnosis, sleep cycles, sleep therapy, external determinants.

The distribution of research articles reflects the trends in this area within and across time. Consistently, across time, almost half of the research has been focused on the internal aspects of sleep—the behavior of the central nervous system, the "wet" systems of endocrinology, biochemistry, and drugs, and the general physiology. Within these areas of interest we can see reflections of the scientific world at work. The drift away from interest in general physiology has reflected both an increased sophistication in our ability to study the central nervous system and a certainty that this is where the fundamental control of sleep is centered. The recent shift from conceiving the central nervous system as a "switchboard" system to seeing it as a "chemical plant" reflects an increased sophistication in biochemical procedures. It also shows that our knowledge about the neurological aspects of sleep has become more fully detailed.

The small rise in the study of sleep disorders and personality variables is an accurate reflection of current trends emphasizing treatment of sleep-related disorders.

The small percentage of effort devoted to dream research, though, is perhaps surprising. This reflects the literature covered and is primarily a report of laboratory studies. As a result the table does not reflect the extensive use of dreams as a clinical tool nor more speculative articles on the meaning of dreams.

This book

From the vast, complex, and growing array of information about sleep we naturally have to make some choices. In this book I am going to concentrate on the psychology of sleep. This means, in the first place, that I will be viewing sleep as a behavior—something we do, an act we perform.

I shall gather together as much data as seems necessary to help us understand and make predictions about this behavior. However, a selection is again necessary. We may try to understand and predict the occurrence and limits of sleep from many levels—for example, from biochemical changes, neurological factors, or cultural conditions. I have chosen to concentrate on the relationships between sleep and "everyday life": those conditions that visibly happen to us from day to day; those that we can recognize and can often do something about. Time, for example: how long we are awake, how long we sleep, when we go to sleep. Age. Noise. Taking or not taking drugs. Dreams that we remember. In short, we are looking at sleep in the environment with which we are most familiar—that of our own daily lives.

The reasonableness of such an enterprise is based upon one fact and an increasing certainty. The fact is that sleeping is a dominant behavior in our lives. It occupies about a third of our earthly doings. Before this behavior all other behaviors bow down each day and year after year of our time. In its presence we "sow not nor do we toil." We leave our labors, our loves, our ambitions, our successes, and our troubled ways. To ignore this massive and dominant behavior is to ignore much of our very existence itself.

The growing certainty is that the nature of this behavior is predictable and understandable. It differs among people. Some people sleep less or more than others. It is done easily or with difficulty. There are literally millions of insomniacs and even more millions who sleep without a thought about their sleep. Sleep is affected by many conditions: when we sleep, how regularly, under what circumstances. Sleep changes dramatically from infancy to old age. Within sleep we dream, sleep lightly or heavily. When we fail to sleep, we behave differently. However, the important point is this: we are increasingly able to predict when these variations are going to occur, and under what circumstances. It becomes clearer and clearer that sleep is not an erratic happenstance but is a remarkably lawful system. If we can know the relationships within this system, we may be able to use them.

This book consists of essentially four parts, each building upon the preceding sections.

The following two chapters (2–3) are descriptions of the dimensions and organization of sleep. How do we measure and describe this hidden world? What's going on in there while we're "away"? It is necessary to know the natural shape and form of the sleep process before we can begin to know its variations.

The next seven chapters (4–10) are reports on and analyses of the variations in sleep. In Chapter 4 the question being asked is what happens to sleep as a person ages? The sleep of infants is vastly different from that of the young or the aged. On the average it is twice as long and occurs in frequent short bursts across the twenty-four hours. We will examine the course of these changes. In Chapter 5 we will consider the effects of varying the timing of sleep. What happens to sleep as we stay up later, arise earlier, take naps, jet to Europe, or become shift workers? Chapter 6 is a review of the effects of day-to-day activities and the sleep environment on the sleeping process. Does sleep differ if we study a lot, play tennis, become sad? How does noise affect sleep? Or sleeping in a motel? Or in pajamas versus in the buff? The material in Chapter 7 points up the wide range of individual differences in sleep. In Chapter 8 unusual sleep patterns such as sleep walking and narcolepsy, or "sleep fits," are described. In Chapter 9 the focus is on the effect of disease on sleep. What are the effects of brain damage? Do people with fever or kidney ailments sleep differently? What is the sleep of schizophrenics like? Chapter 10 is a report on the effects of drugs on sleep. How useful are sleeping pills? What about stimulants? These are some of the questions examined there.

The next two chapters are essentially "results" chapters. In Chapter 11 the insomnias and their treatment are discussed. Chapter 12 is an evaluation of the effect of variations in sleep on behavior. What happens if we go without sleep for several days? Suppose we don't get certain kinds of sleep—what are the consequences?

The last three chapters are special considerations. Chapter 13 is devoted to dreams—their place in sleep and their meaning. The analysis of their meaning will include an attempt to understand not only what their content reflects but also how they function within sleep. In Chapter 14 I will attempt to synthesize the preceding material and to draw a conclusion to the question: why do we sleep? Finally, in Chapter 15 I will try to answer frequently asked questions about sleep which may have eluded our outline; among these will be matters dealing with the relationship of sleep to hypnosis and hibernation, sleep and brainwashing, and sleep learning.

Implications

The dark kingdom of sleep is a curious and mysterious one into which we enter each 24 hours. Until very recently its mysteries have prevailed. However, from laboratories throughout the world, expeditions have been launched and, with increasing efficiency, have brought back more and more information about that hidden world. The explorers have been researchers from a wide range of scientific disciplines. Each, at his or her own level of description, has been trying to help us understand sleep and its place in our lives.

I hope that this book will provide a better understanding of the laws and landscape of that dark kingdom so that we may be more certain of our ways of behaving in relationship to it and within it—so that, indeed, we may be better citizens of the realm of sleep.

2

The dimensions of sleep

We must begin our excursion into the world of sleep by learning its dimensions. Someone has said that science operates on a rule of "measurement before existence." Of course, there are many things that exist which can't be measured very well, or at all: the beauty of a Rembrandt, feelings about death, the twinkle of an eye. But for science measurement is necessary because the scientific endeavor *is* the business of accurately describing, comparing, and relating things to each other. In describing sleep we must do considerably better than to say that it is something we do when we are not awake. This is as of little use as describing death as the state of not being alive.

This chapter and the next are necessary steps in accurately describing what sleep is like. First, we will consider the place of sleep within the 24 hours: amount, length of sleep periods, and placement of sleep. Second, we will look at the internal process of sleep while it is occurring. Then, in the following chapter, we will study the organization of the elements that make up sleep.

The precise measurement of sleep is a technical and detailed affair. I have done my best to minimize the technical aspects. At this point, in books of this type, the author often says something like "Those of you who are interested in the behavior of sleep itself may wish to skip the next two chapters." I cannot so advise you. I believe that from these chapters you will come to know sleep considerably better. More important, you will gain some confidence that the net which we have spread to capture this "whale among fishes" is a sound one.

Sleep within the 24 hours

It is always a surprise to me that, for all of its seemingly complicated ways, sleep varies along only three simple dimensions within the 24 hours. The complex differences in individual patterns of sleep result from there being more or less sleep in the time period and different times of beginning and ending. However, these simple elements of variation can be arranged into quite complex differences.

Sleep length: The length of sleep varies among individuals because some people go to sleep earlier or later than is usual, get up earlier or later, or sleep, on the average, more or less than others. There are also differences within the same person from day to day. The total amount of sleep in 24 hours can be varied, in addition, by adding naps.

Sleep onset and termination: Sleep onset times may be quite regular—for example, in cases where a person goes to bed at about the same time each night—may vary occasionally, or be quite irregular. The degree of irregularity may be great or small: an individual may go to bed sometimes at 11:00 P.M., sometimes at 11:30 P.M., sometimes at 10:00 P.M., and sometimes at 2:00 A.M. Awakening times tend to be somewhat more regular because of work schedules. Sleep onset time may be systematically changed. For example, a person may go on a shift-work schedule.

These changes usually are interactive but may be independent. By holding either onset or arousal time constant but varying one, sleep length is varied. By introducing additional onset times such as naps the number of episodes within 24 hours is changed. However, if both onset and arousal time are shifted in the same direction by the same amount, sleep length is unchanged.

To know about how a person sleeps we must be able to specify, within each 24 hours, the length of each sleep episode and the onset of each sleep episode. From these two measures we can talk about such a variety of topics as infant sleep, shift work, long and short sleepers, jet lag, regular sleepers, sleep deprivation, and the like.

The substructure of sleep

Sleep is not simply a "turning off" or "going flat" or a "nothingness" in which we lie awash. It is a very busy and active state of affairs. This continuous activity occurs at a number of levels and can be described from the perspective of neuroanatomical involvement, biochemical processes, nerve cells, physiological changes (temperature, heart rate, blood pressure), amount and kinds of bodily movements, levels of consciousness, or in more general terms such as "lying down with the eyes closed." We may even describe sleep poetically, for example, "wrapped in the arms of Morpheus." These events, present within sleep, we have labeled as the substructures of sleep.

Each and all such descriptions can be completely accurate and, for particular purposes, useful or necessary. For a complete description of the ongoing sleep process they and a host of other measurements—of glandular changes, blood flow in various body parts, and metabolism, for example—would be necessary. This is obviously not feasible and, for the behavioral study of sleep, not likely to be useful or even critical. What is needed is an index that reflects the major behavioral aspects of sleep.

One such measure has emerged and has come to be the instrument predominantly used in describing or indexing and even defining sleep. This is the electroencephalogram, which measures changes in "brain waves" during sleep. I will first describe these patterns in sleep and then point out their particular usefulness in sleep analyses.

The electroencephalogram

The electroencephalogram (*electro* = "electrical"; *encephalon* = "brain"; *gram* = "record"), which is usually referred to as the EEG, is a writing out on paper of the "brain wave."

The brain wave is a natural property of the brain that reflects a "field" of electrical activity. This activity is in the microvolt range (one-millionth of a volt). While we live, this electrical activity is ever-present. It is a continuously changing field; that is, there is a continuing fluctuation in the voltage level in both frequency and amplitude. This is a reflection, in a complex and not yet understood way, of the electrical activity present in the millions of individual nerve cells that comprise the brain.

Brain waves are measured by attaching conductors to the scalp. These are small cups, about a half inch in diameter, containing a highly conductive paste which is "glued" to the skin. Wires leading from these conductors (gathered into a "pigtail"), go to the EEG machine.

The EEG machine simply amplifies (magnifies) the small electrical potential changes and converts them to a mechanical write-out on a continuously running paper belt. The principle is much the same as that of the record player and its amplifier system, but the conversion there, of course, is to sound.

Looking carefully at the records that result from EEG recordings taken from sleeping subjects, researchers have found five discernible patterns which the wave forms take. These are called "sleep stages."

Figure 2-1 illustrates the five stages of sleep and the waking EEG. Somehow these patterns managed to escape an esoteric nomenclature and are simply labeled Stages 1, 2, 3, 4, and 1-REM. Wakefulness is labeled Stage 0. The highlights or distinguishing characteristics of these patterns are as follows:

Stage 0: This is the waking state just preceding sleep and is identified by the presence of "alpha rhythm," an 8- to 12-cycle-per-second symmetrical wave form.

Stage 1: This stage is characterized by low voltage activity (low amplitude in the electroencephalogram) with a mixed arrhythmic pattern.

Stage 2: This stage is identified by the presence of "sleep spindles," which are very brief bursts (from ½ second to about 2 seconds in duration) of 13- to 16-cycle-per-second waves (identified by arrows in the figure). There are also "K-complexes," which are sharp rises and falls and "recovery" of the EEG. K-complexes occur in the waking subject (without spindles) in response to discrete signal inputs but occur spontaneously in sleep.

Stage 3: This is a transition between Stage 2 and Stage 4 containing both the "slow waves" of Stage 4 and the continuing presence of "spindles" and K-complexes of Stage 2.

Stage 4: Stage 4 is defined as more than 50 percent of the scoring epoch consisting of slow waves of a specified amplitude level. The slow waves range from .5 to 3 cycles per second.

Stage 1-REM: This stage is scored in the presence of a Stage 1 EEG pattern and the presence of "rapid eye movements" (REMs). These eye movements are not continuous but typically occur in short bursts and are generally in the range of one or two movements per second.

The scoring of records is usually done visually by trained scorers in sequential steps of 30-second or 1-minute units. Trained scorers will agree with one another at least 90 percent of the time on the scoring of a night's record.

The organization of these stages within sleep, the variations that occur, and their specific functions will be detailed later. However, a few general comments about the stages need to be made at this point.

The alpha rhythm of Stage 0 is seen only when the person is completely relaxed and not "thinking about or attending to" something. This state of "nonthinking" is, of course, a natural precursor to

FIG. 2-1 EEG tracing of the sleep stages. The records have been reduced to about 50 percent of their actual size.

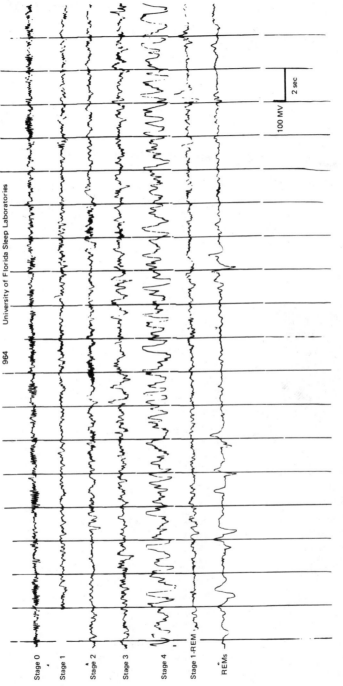

Stage 0

Stage 1

Stage 2

Stage 3

Stage 4

Stage 1-REM

REMs

964   University of Florida Sleep Laboratories

100 MV

2 sec

Source: University of Florida Sleep Laboratories

14 Sleep: The Gentle Tyrant

the drifting off into sleep, and the disappearance of alpha is a good index of sleep onset. However, as soon as the subject begins to concentrate, try to solve a problem, for example, the alpha rhythm disappears and the EEG pattern is not distinguishable from Stage 1 sleep. Furthermore, even in the resting and relaxed state some 20 percent of the population have minimal or no alpha. Both of these factors make scoring of Stage 0 more difficult. Often, for experimental purposes subjects are chosen for good "baseline" alpha rhythms. In addition, the onset of Stage 2 may be used for sleep onset measures (see below). This dual directionality from Stage 0 is sometimes labeled descending Stage 1 (going to sleep) and ascending Stage 1 (alerting). The Stage 1 after sleep onset and associated with Stage 1-REM sleep is generally considered to be the latter rather than a state of "drowsiness."

With good alpha subjects the measurement of the onset of sleep by the EEG is quite accurate. This can be best seen in a study done in our laboratory. We had subjects attempt to go to sleep within a 45-minute period at 10:00 A.M. after a full night's sleep. We used this condition as a maximally difficult set of records to score since the subjects may or may not have been able to go to sleep and the length of time required to go to sleep would be more variable than would be typical after a full day of wakefulness. Two scorers scored the records for the appearance of Stage 1 and of Stage 2. The scorers agreed perfectly that 39 percent of the records showed no "spindles" (Stage 2) and that 17 percent did not reach Stage 1. In short, there was perfect agreement about the subjects that did not sleep. For the records showing sleep onset, the two scorers set the sleep onset time within two minutes of each other eight times out of ten using either Stage 1 or Stage 2. Only 3 percent of the Stage 2 and 9 percent of the Stage 1 scored records times disagreed by more than five minutes. There was, then, good agreement as to whether sleep had occurred or not and, when it occurred, differences in onset times were quite small.

Again, recognizing that these tests of the measures were made under most difficult conditions for scoring, we can interpret this study to mean that sleep onset can be effectively measured by the EEG.

Do these measures actually measure the process of going to sleep? In the same experiment we asked half the subjects after the 45-minute period whether they "had gone to sleep." Table 2-1 shows the comparison of their answers to the sleep stage actually reached during the 45-minute period.

It is difficult to understand the answer of "No" or "Don't Know" to the stages of certain sleep (Stages 3/4). Perhaps the same incomprehensible factor accounts for the few subjects who responded "No" or

TABLE 2-1   Sleep Stage Attained

	0	1	2	3-4
"I went to sleep"		40%	85%	90%
"I didn't sleep"	100%	60%	10%	5%
"I don't know"			5%	5%

"Don't Know" to Stage 2. Generally, however, the presence of Stage 2 was coordinate with perceived sleep. The Stage 1 responses indicate that this is indeed a very light stage of sleep. However, it is possible that a few of the "No"-responding subjects may have been actually in "ascending Stage 1" and actively thinking about something.

After the onset of sleep, Stages 1 through 4 have been shown to be generally related to the depth of sleep when depth of sleep is defined as "arousability" or "responsiveness to external stimulation." This relationship is discussed in some detail in Chapter 6.

Stage 1-REM has been studied more intensively than the other stages of sleep because of its many unique aspects. Among the most prominent of these is the clear association between this stage of sleep and dream content. We will detail this relationship in Chapter 13.

Because of the presence of dreams and a number of other different characteristics associated with Stage 1-REM sleep when compared with the rest of the sleep period and waking, there has been a tendency to view this as a "third state." Certainly it is a condition that we will find central in all of our continuing considerations.

Finally, let me make mention here of a particularly important and fortunate aspect of the EEG relative to sleep. I have described above the responsiveness of the EEG to the presence of human sleep. Sleep may be similarly defined or measured in animals. Clear-cut EEG changes have been demonstrated with the onset of sleep and stages of sleep have been found in essentially all mammals and even in birds. The major differences are that below the primates (monkeys and apes) the sleep is generally confined to two stages—a slow-wave sleep (Stage 4) and a Stage 1-REM sleep—and the timing between REM episodes is shorter.

The EEG as a good measure of sleep

As noted earlier, the ongoing process of sleep involves a complex interaction of phenomena that has been described along many dimensions. The earliest systematic work in the 1870s tried to measure sleep "depth" by testing subjects' sensitivities to varying stimuli throughout the night. Motility, or body movements, began to be explored starting in the early 1900s and was still a factor in Russian research under the name of "actographs" into the 1960s. In the 1930s various physiological measures such as temperature, heart rate, breathing, and electrodermal levels were pursued as correlates of sleep. Today the substructural events of single nerve cells, neurophysiological systems, biochemical, and endocrine changes can also be determined. Throughout, the subject's own descriptions of his sleep have also been assayed. Why has the EEG emerged as essentially the prime descriptor of the substructure of sleep?

We can best answer this by asking what the general requirements of a good process measure are and applying these to the various measures. The following eight characteristics are among the more obvious:

1. Does not interfere with the process being measured
2. Can be applied without excessive technical or expense demands
3. Is continuous throughout the process
4. Shows promising discriminable subcategories
5. Utilizable across a wide range of subjects and conditions
6. Correlates with other major components of the process
7. Stable across similar conditions
8. Sensitive across varied conditions

Clearly the EEG is the only measure that comes close to meeting these criteria satisfactorily. It does not wake the subject up. It is not excessive in technical and expense demands (although it is not exactly simple or inexpensive). It is continuous and can yield a second-by-second picture of sleep. It has discriminable categories. It is useful, for example, in small animals such as mice as well as in larger creatures such as humans, and can be telemetered from orbiting space stations. It correlates with such variables as sleep onset, depth of sleep, and dreams. It produces a similar pattern of sleep from night to night under similar conditions. It will be the point of much of this text to track its sensitivity to varied conditions. All of the earlier explored measures fail one or more of the criteria outlined.

Small wonder that this measuring instrument has served sleep research so well. It is certainly an advance on the measurement system used in the sleep world of Dr. Seuss.

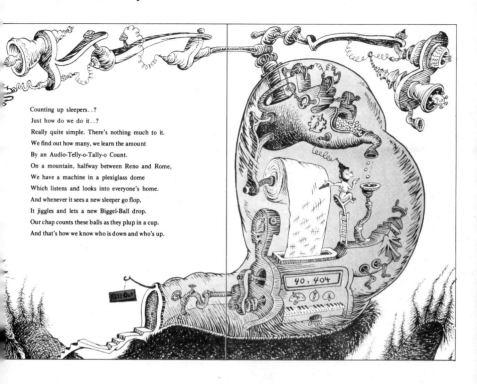

Counting up sleepers..?
Just how do we do it..?
Really quite simple. There's nothing much to it.
We find out how many, we learn the amount
By an Audio-Telly-o-Tally-o Count.
On a mountain, halfway between Reno and Rome,
We have a machine in a plexiglass dome
Which listens and looks into everyone's home.
And whenever it sees a new sleeper go flop,
It jiggles and lets a new Biggel-Ball drop.
Our chap counts these balls as they plup in a cup.
And that's how we know who is down and who's up.

Summary and implications

We have laid the groundwork for describing sleep and its variations by describing the major dimensions of the process. We divided sleep into the variables describing its place within the 24 hours and the variations occurring within the state itself. These are the basic elements of sleep.

By attending to length and onset times of sleep episodes and the resultant covariants—amount, diurnal placement, and number of episodes—we can effectively "reproduce" or describe any pattern of sleep that may occur in a 24-hour period.

We have further described the changes in the EEG associated with sleep that permit a moment-to-moment description of what is going on during sleep.

We are now ready to move to the organization of these variables.

3

The organization of sleep

As we move through this book we shall see that there are immense variations in sleeping from time to time in our own sleep and among individuals. Each individual sleeps more or less and at different times. Some individuals sleep more or less than others. Infants sleep differently from the aged, and animals sleep differently from each other. Sleep differs under varying conditions: drugs, noise, shift work, illnesses, and weekends all affect it. Some people sleep poorly and others well. There are sleep variants such as sleepwalking. Within sleep, stages shift in amount and timing in a complex dance. The bulk of this book will be concerned with these many variations.

To understand them, however, we must first know what "natural" or "normal" sleep is like. We must know what "unvaried" sleep is before we can know how or, indeed, whether a particular sleep pattern is significant in its differences. We can make this comparison in two general ways. We can measure the sleep of an individual or group of individuals under "normal" conditions and compare these measurements to the sleep under "different" circumstances. We do this in experiments. We first measure the "normal" sleep and then, for example, give a drug or introduce some stress and see if there has been a change. Often, however, we have reason to believe that the individual's sleep will vary from the "normal," due to some physical or mental condition; he is perhaps a chronic alcoholic or a bed wetter, and we want to know if and how his sleep is distorted or different from the norm. In these circumstances we would compare his sleep to that of individuals who were "normal"; that is, were similar to the individual except that they were not alcoholic or bed wetters.

There is a complication. Can we describe "normal" sleep in such a way that we can compare sleep under varied conditions? To do this we must examine the complex patterns of sleep to determine if there are common and stable patterns in the organization of normal sleep that can permit us to "index" or describe it. This is what I will try to do here.

For the purposes of obtaining an "anchor point" to describe the properties of normal sleep we have chosen the sleep of normal young adults. We have chosen this group as our anchor point because theirs is the simplest and most common form of sleep, which holds in general terms between the early teens and the mid and late thirties. By normal young adults we simply mean individuals who report no physical complaints nor show any apparent psychological deviations. They are between 18 and 22 years of age, have no complaints about their sleep, and are not heavy drug users. Much of the data reported in this chapter comes from our laboratories at the University of Florida. The EEG data is from subjects who reported to the laboratory at 10:00 P.M., were wired for recordings, and slept from about 11:00 P.M. to 7:00 A.M. for four successive nights. The data on sleep length and placement was collected from two-week sleep logs filled out by the students.

The organization of sleep and waking

Young-adult sleep is generally organized into one long sleep period of about seven to eight hours during the night. A general exception to this general pattern is the presence of a once-a-day nap in some people and some populations. In many subtropical cultures, for instance, an afternoon nap or "siesta" is the norm rather than the exception. There is, however, a remarkable and often not noticed variability around this general pattern both between and within individuals.

Approached casually the question of sleep length in the young adult would seem to be quite simple. If you were asked "How long do people sleep?" your answer most likely would be, "Oh, about seven or eight hours." While there is some truth in this very general answer, it is not true of all people all the time nor of some people some of the time. This is particularly pertinent in regard to college students, who are less bound by regular work hours and more battered by varied class and work schedules, social growth problems and pleasures, and varied academic requirements.

A group of 89 students, 47 males and 42 females, completed a sleep log in which they carefully recorded their sleep and waking times over several weeks. Some of the highlights of these logs were as follows.

Sleep length:
—The average sleep length at night was 7 hours and 40 minutes.
—The average sleep amount per 24 hours—including naps—was 8 hours and 5 minutes.
—The average amount of sleep per 24 hours for the shortest sleeper was 6 hours and 5 minutes and for the longest sleeper was 9 hours and 55 minutes.
—Only 51 percent of the subjects averaged between 7 and 8 hours per night on the average.
—The average subject had 66 percent of his nightly sleep lengths falling in a 3-hour range, with 95 percent of his nightly lengths in a 6-hour range. One subject, however, had a sleep length that ranged from 0.0 hours to 11 hours and 5 minutes.
—The average length of sleep of the subjects on weekdays was 7 hours and 25 minutes, while the average length of sleep on weekends was 8 hours and 20 minutes.

The placement of sleep: In a theoretical picture of young-adult sleep, with the exception of the siesta cultures, the presumed "normal" pattern would be a single sleep period, occurring at a relatively fixed onset and arousal time. The data from our college students belies this simplistic scheme. Across a two-week period:
—The amount of napping was far greater than expected: No naps = 16 percent; 1–2 naps = 26 percent; 3–4 naps = 16 percent; 5 or more = 42 percent.
—The regularity of going to bed and getting up varied. Only 3 percent went to bed within a half hour of the same time each night. Three percent varied by as much as three hours earlier or later than their average during the two-week period.
—Getting up was somewhat more regular. Two percent got up within a half hour of their average wakeup time most mornings, but 7 percent varied by more than 2 hours during a two week period.
—The time of going to bed was also varied. The average time of going to bed was 12:45 A.M., but 6 percent went to bed before 11 P.M. on the average while 9 percent went to bed on the average after 2:00 A.M.
—The average time of getting up was 8:25 A.M. Four percent got up before 7:00 A.M. while 6 percent got up after 10:00 A.M. on the average.
While we recognize that these students undoubtedly show an unusual picture of sleep and waking because of the particular circumstances under which they are operating, the variability is impressive and the picture of the superstructure of sleep that is reflected is far from simple. Within these relatively self-selected

schedules of individuals who can be presumed to be functioning with a reasonable degree of effectiveness, the range of patterning is provocative. The total amount of sleep within 24 hours, while averaging close to 8 hours, had a range of 4 (6.1–9.9) hours. The length of sleep varied from night to night for each subject and between weekdays and week-ends. The placement of sleep also showed variability in the regularity of going to bed and getting up and the particular time chosen. The pure uniphasic pattern of sleep (without naps) was maintained by only 16 percent of the subjects.

In passing, we would note and answer a rather natural question about these data. About half the subjects were male and about half were female. There were essentially no differences in their sleep characteristics. We shall have several occasions to return to this finding.

The data on naps is particularly provocative in relation to the presumed character of the superstructure of sleep. How natural is the uniphasic pattern under which we "typically" operate and certainly assume to be the norm? We shall see that the nap is the last element to be maintained in the restructuring of infant sleep into adult sleep and shows a strong resurgence in the advancing years. Further, in many subtropical and tropical regions the noonday siesta and resultant biphasic pattern is the normative sleep pattern. In "time-free" environments in which subjects are permitted "ad libitum" schedules of sleep and waking, half the subjects displayed clearly discernible nap patterns.

Above all, the data on length and placement emphasizes, for better or worse, the very real presence of large between-person and within-person variations that are a part of the nature of sleep.

The organization within sleep

Let us begin by "writing out" the sleep of a young man who was recorded in the laboratory during three nights. These three nights, using minute-by-minute sleep-stage scores, are shown in Figure 3-1. The lower line for each night is divided into hours and begins with the young man's going to bed. Each sleep stage is given across these sleep periods. REM sleep is designated by solid bars.

From these figures one can get a good picture of each night of sleep. For example, on the first night the subject was awake for about 5 minutes and step by step went through Stages 1, 2, 3, and 4, arriving at Stage 4 sleep about 25 minutes after retiring. He briefly dropped back to Stage 2 and returned to Stage 4, and after about 80 minutes

Fɪɢ. 3-1   The sleep stages of a single subject sleeping for three successive nights in the laboratory. Stages are given on the vertical and hours from the time in bed are on the horizontal. The black bars indicate periods of REM sleep.

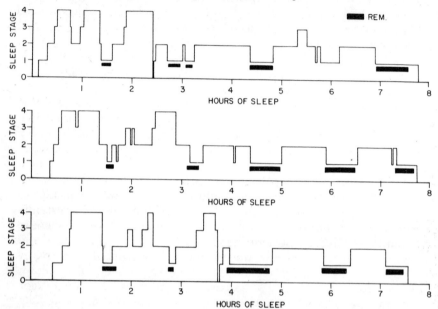

Source: Progress in Clinical Psychology, eds. L. E. Abt and B. P. Riess (New York: Grune & Stratton, Inc., 1969), Fig. 2, p. 17. Used by permission.

there was a burst of REM sleep of about 10 minutes. He then returned to deep sleep and awakened briefly in the second hour. There was an interrupted REM episode before awakening. On the second night he was awake for about 15 minutes, went more quickly to Stage 4 sleep, briefly dropped into Stage 3, returned to Stage 4, and after about 90 minutes had a brief REM episode. There was a later Stage 4 period and the second REM episode was delayed until the third hour. There were then 3 succeeding REM episodes. The third night showed again a similar but slightly different pattern of sleep when compared to the first two.

By writing out his sleep stages in this manner, we can certainly know a great deal about this young man's sleep on these three nights. There is a difficulty, however. Suppose this had been an experiment in which, for example, we had been studying the effect of stress on sleep and nights one and three had been control (nonstress) nights and night 2 had been the night before a crucial examination (the stress night). It would be difficult by looking at these complex changes to tell whether stress had had an effect. Clearly we need some way to further encode these nights of sleep to see if there was a difference between nights.

Two of the most effective and common ways of summarizing and analyzing the sleep substructure for comparative purposes have been through the study of total sleep stages and temporal relationships during sleep.

Total sleep stages

Table 3-1 presents the total sleep-stage percentages for the three nights of our example, the averages of three night records for 30 young adults and the associated standard deviations and, as a contrasting set of data, the three-night averages of a 60-year-old subject. These sleep-stage amounts are given in percentages of total sleep time since this has the effect of minimizing differences in sleep length. The standard deviations are a measure of variability around the average; about 2/3 of all the scores fall within one standard deviation above or below the average and nearly all scores fall within three standard deviations above and below the average.

TABLE 3-1   Average Percentages of Total Sleep Stages

	0	1	2	3	4	REM
Figure 3-1, Night 1	2	12	47	6	16	19
Night 2	0	7	48	3	15	26
Night 3	0	10	43	7	13	27
Young adults (18–22)	1	5	48	7	15	24
Sixty-year-olds	9	12	51	5	3	21
Young adults' standard deviations	1	2	5	2	5	4

This table can tell us a great deal about the organization of sleep stages and about our particular subject. First, the group data tells us that sleep stages are organized in mini-maxi "bands" around different characteristic amounts for each stage. The following limits are "built in" as the boundaries of each sleep stage: Very few "normal" young adults exceed these limits.

Stage 0	=	0% to 3%
Stage 1	=	1% to 10%
Stage 2	=	40% to 60%
Stage 3	=	3% to 12%
Stage 4	=	5% to 25%
REM	=	15% to 35%

This data is saying that sleep is "programmed" to go through these stages and sets of limits each night. No one is a "Stage 4 sleeper" or a

"REM" sleeper during a full night. Rather, in young adults there will seldom be more than 24 percent Stage 4 sleep and seldom less than 12 percent Stage 4 sleep, and there will seldom be more than 30 percent REM sleep or less than 15 percent REM sleep.

Now let's look at our example. First, we can see that he is a "normal" sleeper since his percentages fall well within the average and range of his age group. Second, notice that he shows a consistency in his sleep from night to night. He is consistently higher in his Stage 1 sleep amount, for example, since he is toward the upper end of the range. Third, we can now say that if other subjects acted in a similar manner and Night 2 had been an experimental night, the variable— in this case, stress—was not an important factor in affecting sleep, since Night 2 showed little difference in sleep-stage amounts.

However, look at the 60-year-old subject. This example informs us of the sensitivity of the particular measure used, since the patterns show clear-cut deviations from the young adults in a sharply reduced Stage 4 and an increased Stage 0 and 1.

Temporal aspects

Look back at Figure 3-1. You will notice that on these three nights sleep stages 3 and 4 tended to occur early in the night. You will also see that REM sleep (the solid bar) does not occur within the first hour and tends to become greater in amount as the sleep period progresses. These are important and consistent features of the organization of sleep which can be used to determine whether significant changes have occurred in a particular sleep period. Figure 3-2 has plotted the hour by hour amount of Stage 4 and REM sleep for the 30 subjects whose amount data was reported in the Table 3-1 above.

Notice that by this measure we can say that the subject in our example has a "normal temporal" distribution of his sleep, since it shows generally the same distribution as that of his age group—early Stage 4 sleep and increasing REM sleep.

These temporal measures add great sensitivity to our ability to assess the effects that varied conditions have on sleep. For example, Figure 3-3 shows the distribution of Stages 4 and REM across a sleep period for a group of subjects who were required to sleep from 8:00 A.M. to 4:00 P.M. instead of 11:00 P.M. to 7:00 A.M. This is what happens to sleep when a person goes on shift work. Clearly the temporal order of sleep is sharply changed when it is compared to Figure 3-2. REM sleep occurs earlier and with considerable vigor, and

Fig. 3-2 The hourly distribution of minutes of Stage 4 and Stage REM sleep across an 8-hour sleep period. The average results from 30 young adult subjects.

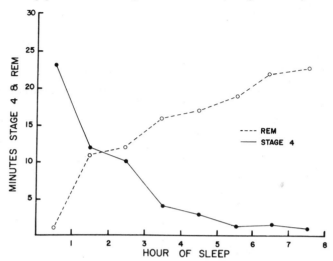

is depressed later in sleep. Stage 4 is depressed initially and is extended into a later time.

We shall discuss the more general effects of shift work in the next

Fig. 3-3 The hourly distribution of the minutes of Stage 4 and REM sleep when sleep occurs during the day. These are the averages of six subjects who typically slept from 11:00 P.M. to 7:00 A.M.

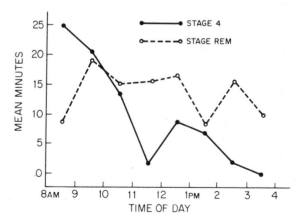

Source: Figure 2, p. 484 of *Chronobiology*, eds. L. E. Scheving, J. E. Pauly, and F. Halberg (Tokyo: Igaku Shoin Ltd.).

chapter, but here this figure can be also used to emphasize the "wisdom" of the sleep system. The total amount of REM and Stage 4 sleep under this "shift" differs little from that occurring in its regular time interval. While REM occurred early, the amount "eased" off in the later period and Stage 4 showed a similarly "balanced" picture. This emphasizes the "programmed" power of this dynamic system.

REM sleep is usually analyzed, in addition to total amount, in terms of its "cycling," which is an appearance of REM episodes in intervals of about 90 minutes. Each "burst" becomes longer, which results in the increasing amount of REM across sleep time (Figure 3-1). Because of this there is a typical report of the latency of REM (time between sleep onset and the first REM episode), the interval between REM episodes, and the length of REM episodes.

Other substructure measures

Again returning to Figure 3-1, you will notice that there are a large number of shifts from stage to stage across the night and that these shifts generally follow a consistent order. The average number of stage changes during a night for young adults is about 35. The order of changes from Stage 1 to Stage 4 is from one serially numbered change to the next; from 1 to 2 to 3 to 4 or from 4 to 3 or 2 to 1, etc. It is rare, once sleep has begun and is not interrupted, that a stage is "skipped," for instance, from 1 to 4 or 4 to 2. REM typically emerges from Stage 2. Both the number of changes per night and the serial order are sometimes used as an assessment variable.

There is an increasing tendency in research to "subanalyze" aspects of the sleep stages. REM sleep, for example, is by no means a period of constant eye movements. Rather, they tend to occur in "bursts" of different "densities" (eye movements per minute), with as much as five minutes between such bursts. These may vary from person to person and from condition to condition. For example, it has been found that "nonrecallers" of dreams have fewer eye movements per unit time than those who recall many dreams. Other submeasures being investigated are the number of "spindles" in Stage 2 per unit time and the appearance of transient bursts of "alpha" or "spindles" within Stage 4 or REM. There is, for example, some indication that "high" alpha within sleep may be a particular form of insomnia.

Implications

Sleep has natural and stable qualities. While varying from time to time within and between individuals, these organizational properties are so fundamental that they permit us to know when an individual's sleep is disturbed or is showing unusual responsiveness to imposed conditions.

The measures of sleep within the 24 hours, while variable, over sufficient periods of time show individual stability. In young adults the length of sleep is heavily centered around seven to eight hours although consistent patterns of sleep of from six to nine and a half hours are present. Typically, within our Western culture, a single nighttime episode of sleep in 24 hours is the norm. In "free time" schedules, naps occur with a surprisingly high frequency. However, when naps are persistent, prolonged, or multiple, one looks more carefully.

The substructure measures of sleep are at once more fixed and more sensitive. They are certainly almost totally independent of self-control and are essentially "programmed" processes. The stages of sleep occur within certain narrow limits of amount and each individual sleeps typically within these limits. Further, the stages are organized in timed sequences in their occurrence across sleep periods. We may use significant variations in sleep-stage amounts or placement as signs of disturbed or modified sleep.

4

The changes with age

The patterns of sleep are dramatically affected by the certain fact that we grow older. As one researcher put it, the differences in sleep between age levels "far exceed in magnitude those produced by any pathological condition compatible with life." Because of the magnitude of these changes, and because the process of aging is inevitable in all our lives and those of our children, we begin our description of the variations in sleep patterns with the changes that occur as a natural consequence of aging.

The sleep of the newborn is, of course, very different from that of young adults. There is almost twice as much of it on the average. It occurs in six or more relatively short bursts scattered across the 24 hours. The substructure is dominated by REM sleep. In the first year there is a reduction in the amount of sleep and a radical redistribution of the patterns of sleep. The long night sleep begins to take shape along with one or two naps. REM sleep amounts begin to decline. In the early years, sleep continues to shift toward the pattern of adulthood. In the forties, changes in the substructure are most prominent, with the diminishing of deep sleep (Stage 4) and increases in awakening (Stage 0) and light sleep (Stage 1). In the late ages, naps are resurgent and nighttime awakenings are more frequent. Throughout this process individual differences are prominent.

We will focus our particular attention on the three periods of most prominent change: the first 6 months, early childhood from the years 1 to 5, and the aging of sleep beyond the thirties.

This chapter is somewhat burdened with numbers. I found this necessary for two reasons. I wanted to emphasize individual differences, and these matters of degree are best seen in specific numbers rather than vaguely qualifying statements such as ". . . but some children do this more or less than others." Further, and perhaps more important, one can only compare effectively with specifics. Wonder, and sometimes even fright, can most often be reduced by comparing our behavior with others. I hope, then, that these specific figures will be useful in reducing our wonder or concern about our own sleep or that of our children—or they may serve to point up problems that deserve attention.

The sleep of infants

Both observational and EEG studies agree in classifying the sleep of the newborn into the categories of "quiet sleep" and "active sleep." In quiet sleep the infant lies without movement except for occasional sudden "startle-like" movements that do not awaken or disturb the infant. The EEG shows bursts of large-amplitude slow waves along with fast, mixed, and low-amplitude waves. During active sleep the child has frequent and continuous movements: the head is often moving from side to side, there is irregular and fast respiration and heart rate, grimaces, and frequent and rapid eye movements that are easily observable. The eyes may even be partially open. During active sleep the EEG shows a distinctly different pattern of low-amplitude arrhythmic waves and no slow waves.

Clearly this active sleep phase shares much in common with the more fully developed REM sleep in maturity. It appears rhythmically, although the cycle is about 60 minutes compared to the 90-minute cycle of the adult. Because the sleep episodes are irregular in occurrence these events may begin at sleep onset. The amount of active sleep is very large in the newborn, ranging from 50 percent to 80 percent. It is proportionally even higher in the premature baby.

Major changes occur in the substructure of sleep in the first year. The amount of active sleep diminishes to about 30 percent in the second six months of life. In addition, the "spindles" that identify the presence of Stage 2 sleep appear in the second month and are typically fully developed in the second six-month period.

Equally dramatic and more apparent are the changes taking place in the distribution of sleep. We are fortunate in having two excellent studies of the patterns of sleep in early infancy. Forty-six infants were observed by mothers from the first week through the sixteenth week and reported on by Parmalee and his associates in 1964. The sleep of nineteen infants during their first 26 weeks was reported by Kleitman and Engelmann in 1953. The studies are in remarkable agreement.

Both studies, conducted on normal, healthy babies, emphasize the individual differences present. For example, Parmalee reports that the average total sleep per 24 hours during the first week was 16.3 hours. However, the range of total sleep for 68 percent of his group of infants was from about 14 to 18 hours. The full range of sleep in the observed infants was from about 11 to 21½ hours per 24-hour period. Notice that one-third of the infants slept more than 18 hours or less than 14 hours. By the sixteenth week, while the average had gone down to 14.8 hours, one-third were sleeping less than 13½ hours or more than 16 hours. Kleitman's data also found these differences. Across his observation period from 3 to 26 weeks, one of his infants averaged 11.8 hours per 24-hour period while another averaged 16.3 hours.

Regarding the changes in total sleep time, Table 4-1 presents the

TABLE 4-1   Total Sleep Each Day (hours)

Age (Weeks)	Parmalee (Average)	Parmalee (Middle 2/3)	Kleitman (Average)
1	16.3	14–18	
2	16.2	14–18	
4	15.4	13–17	14.8
8	15.4	14–17	14.5
12	15.1	13–17	15.0
16	14.8	13–16	14.5
20			14.2
24			13.6
26			13.7

average amounts of sleep per 24 hours for the two groups along with the approximate ranges reported in the Parmalee study. At the end of one month there has been about a 1-hour reduction, by the fourth month about 1½ hours, and by the sixth month about 2 hours per 24 hours of sleep. When we recognize that sleep amount will stabilize in adulthood at about 8 hours of sleep, we can see that some 25 percent of the total change in sleep amount has occurred during this first six months.

Even more dramatic changes occur in the distribution of sleep during this period of life. These changes take two forms: a lengthening of sleep episodes and increasing tendency for sleep to occur at night.

Figure 4-1, taken from Parmalee, shows the average length of the longest sleep period each 24 hours (which we will see is increasingly associated with the night period), the average length of the longest waking period, and the associated changes in total sleep time from birth to 16 weeks. While total sleep time has shown a decrease of 9

FIG. 4-1 The total sleep per 24 hours and the averages of the longest periods of wakefulness and sleep each day within 16 weeks of observation. Data from 46 infants.

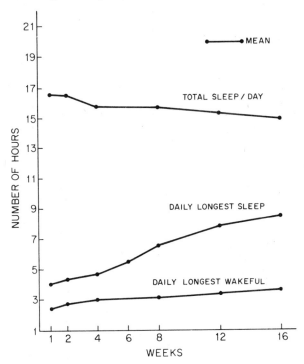

Source: Figure 1, p. 579 of A. H. Parmalee, Jr., W. H. Wenner, and H. R. Schulz, "Infant Sleep Patterns: From Birth to 16 Weeks of Age," *Journal of Pediatrics*, vol. 65, no. 4, 1964, 576–82.

percent and the average tendency to sustain wakefulness has increased by 40 percent (from 2.4 hours to 3.6 hours), the average longest sleep length has more than doubled (from 4.1 to 8.5 hours). With this lengthening of the sleep period there is, of course, a decrease in the number of sleep episodes. In the newborn there will be an average of six to eight sleep periods. As the sleep periods begin to consolidate these will diminish to three to four by the sixth month, with a typical pattern of a long night period, a morning nap, and an afternoon nap.

Perhaps the change in the sleep of the infant most welcomed by parents is seen in the increased nocturnal placement of sleep. Combining the data of Parmalee and Kleitman we find that the average amount of sleep occurring during the night (7:00 P.M. to 7:00 A.M.) and the day (7:00 A.M. to 7:00 P.M.) changes rapidly. In the first week about an equal amount of sleep occurs at night and during the day; 51 percent at night, 49 percent during the day. When we note that in adults night sleep is essentially 100 percent of the sleep time, the sharp increase from 51 percent to 74 percent of the sleep occurring during the night by the end of six months is indeed remarkable. At two months about 50 percent of the infants are awakening during the night at least once, but by the sixth month about 80 percent are sleeping through the night. Stated otherwise, for anxious mothers, about one child in five is continuing to awaken during the night by the sixth month.

One of the early acute observers of infant sleep was Dr. Arnold Gesell. He divided sleep up into four phases: going to sleep, staying asleep, waking up, and staying awake. Before the age of about 16 weeks the infant is not skillful in any of these, though he is best at sleeping. He often falls asleep while nursing, after an intermittent onset. He may awaken crying. He neither stays awake nor asleep for long intervals. However, by 16 weeks there is increasing competence in all four phases. He finishes his meal before he falls asleep, falls asleep effectively, stays asleep, and stays awake for longer and longer stretches and awakens without crying.

Sleep in the preschool ages

Sleep behavior between the ages of one and six years poses "problems" for parents. In a recent survey of 48 mothers of 2-year-old children, 27 percent reported current worries about the sleep of their children and an additional 19 percent acknowledged having had worries in the past. One can guess that a significant portion of these worries stems from four factors. First, the sleep patterns continue to change dramatically during this period, with widespread individual differences in amount and rate of change. Second, some of the sleep anomalies such as night terrors and sleepwalking begin within this span (these will be discussed in Chapter 8). Third, the child is increasingly becoming a social phenomenon and as a result the parental needs and wishes become more prominent. Finally, the parents are almost without information and their expectancies are guided more by guesswork, hope, and convenience than by the child's actual behavior.

There is little change in the substructure of nighttime sleep during this period. There are only two significant differences between two-

and four-year-olds: the four-year-olds have less Stage 1 and longer REM cycles. From a comparison of the substructures of two-year-olds and young adults, with the exception of a significantly higher REM amount (which may simply reflect the longer sleep length), the substructure of sleep seems to have become organized and stabilized before the second year.

The patterns of sleep and waking, however, show clear-cut changes. Table 4-2 uses the data from three studies conducted in the 1930s from nursery school observations to display the total sleep and the daytime sleep occurring during the ages from two to five.

TABLE 4-2 Average Hours of Total Sleep and Naps

Age	Total Sleep	Range	Day-time Sleep	Range
2	$12\frac{1}{4}$ h	$11-13\frac{1}{4}$ h	$1\frac{1}{2}$ h	1–2 h
3	$11\frac{1}{2}$ h	$10\frac{1}{2}-12\frac{1}{2}$ h	$1\frac{1}{4}$ h	1–2 h
4	$11\frac{1}{4}$ h	$10\frac{1}{2}-12$ h	1 h	$\frac{1}{4}-1\frac{1}{2}$ h
5	11 h	$10-11\frac{1}{2}$ h	$\frac{1}{2}$ h	0–1 h

The picture is an extension of the changes begun in the first year. The average amount of sleep by the second year has declined by nearly an hour and a half from the sixth month and will gradually continue to decline by about another hour in the next years. Again the most dramatic changes are seen in the placement of sleep. Night sleep is becoming consolidated. About 25 percent of the two-year-olds are sleeping consistently throughout the night while 25 percent continue to awaken most nights. The nap periods are consolidating into a single nap and diminishing in length, but with a wide range of individual differences. One study reported that at the age of two, 8 percent of children are napping only irregularly, two-thirds have moved to a single nap period, while 25 percent are still taking two or more naps. By the third year only 10 percent of the children are napping each day, and by the fourth year almost none nap daily. In another study a similar pattern was noted. The proportion of children having no nap period rose successively from the age of two to five: 8 percent, 12 percent, 36 percent, and 95 percent respectively. These changes are clearly reflected in Table 4-2. While night sleep remains essentially stable in length, daytime sleep is showing a continuous decline.

Aside from the sleep anomalies (Chapter 10), most of the "problems" of sleep center around attempts to maintain the nap period and in getting the child to sleep. While in theory a nap is often believed to be "good" for the child and certainly helpful to the mother, the difficulty in putting it into practice results from a simple failure to recognize a natural maturational process. Difficulties in getting the child to sleep reflect either simple failures of common sense or conflicts between the parents' needs and the child's.

Going to sleep easily for either the child or the adult involves a disengagement from ongoing activities and a need to sleep. We frequently fail the child on both of these counts. We often expect the child to disengage himself from "roughhousing" with Daddy, replaying his day, or continuing his play. We launch him into bed for our own conveniences of cocktails, eating, or conversation. There clearly needs to be a gradual cooling down and separation from excitement and engagement in order for sleep to be accepted as a more reasonable activity. Sometimes the problem is compounded or caused by a lack of need to sleep on the part of the child. We may have company, or a baby-sitter, or just be exhausted by our child's boundless energy. On such nights the dictum of the author Emerson is too true: "There never was a child so lovely but his mother was glad to get him to sleep." Sometimes the problem is a firmly held belief about how much sleep the child needs, which may differ markedly from the child's own need. When the child has no need to sleep, our desires are less likely to create the need than a problem.

A question often asked is "How long should my child sleep?" I refer you back to Table 4-2. Sleep amounts vary as greatly as three hours among individual children. My general answer is, "Wake the child up at the same time every morning and watch the child at nighttime." When the puzzled response is, "But I asked you how long my child should sleep," I reply, "I can't answer you, but your child can."

If the child is awakened every morning at the same time, sleep has a chance of consistently raising its signals of need both in regard to naps and to bedtime. Admittedly the signals may not be simple, since they must struggle against the wishes to continue to play, or to remain with the parents, or to "be grown up," or simply not to miss anything. However, the signs of the struggle will be there and a fully awake child should not be forced to bed and a sleepy child needs help in his struggle.

The teens and young adulthood

The natural changes in sleep beyond the age of six and into our thirties are generally unremarkable. The total amount of sleep continues to show a gradual decline from the years 6 to 16 from about 11 hours to about 8 hours. The pattern is essentially a uniphasic nocturnal one. In the superstructure the major change is in the amount of Stage 1-REM sleep, which declines from about 30 percent to 25 percent by the age of 12.

As seen in our previous chapter, variations between and within individuals are clearly present. However, except for the differences in total sleep amounts most of the variations appear to be our own creations imposed upon a largely stable system. These imposed variations will be the topics of our next several chapters.

1881104

The sleep of the aging

As one moves from the thirties into the "golden years" (the writer has entered his fifties, hence the euphemism), the substructure of sleep begins a course of accelerating changes which clearly break through into the patterns of sleep and waking. This pattern has evidence of a "fraying" and diminishing control of the sleep process.

If you will refer back to Table 3-1 of the previous chapter you will find a comparison of the sleep of a young adult population with that of a 60-year-old group. You will see that dramatic changes have taken place with aging. The amount of time awake after sleep onset (Stage 0) has increased ninefold. The number of such awakenings has increased from an average of 1 per night to 6 per night. Light sleep (Stage 1) is two and a half times as great in the 60-year-old. While REM sleep and Stage 2 sleep have shown little change, deep sleep (Stage 4) has diminished markedly by from 15 percent to 30 percent.

There are wide individual differences in the response of sleep to age. Some individuals, more fortunate than others, show little change in their sleep patterns. For example, although the average number of awakenings was six, about 20 percent had no awakenings, while others had ten or more. In an intensive study of sixteen 50-year-old males, four had no deep sleep while three had the amounts of Stage 4 typically present in 30-year-olds.

Most studies have reflected a difference between men and women in regard to the aging process of sleep. The sleep of women is, in general, more resistant to age changes. One study found the sleep of 60-year-old women essentially 10 years "younger" than the sleep of men of the same age, resembling that of men in their fifties rather than in their sixties.

These changes in the substructure of sleep as seen in the laboratory are clearly reflected in self-reports about sleep. Sleep diaries were kept by 40 persons each in the decades between 20 and 60 years of age. The number of during-the-night awakenings reported steadily rose across the decades and was five times greater in the 60-year-old group as compared with the 20-year-old group. Oddly, when compared with the substructure data, the women reported twice the number of awakenings and also reported more sleep disturbances than the men.

Studies consistently report little change in the length of sleep until the sixties. At this point most studies report a slight rise in the average amount of sleep per 24 hours. This picture is, of course, complicated by changes in life-style such as retirement, and physical ailments. What is clear from most studies is that, while the overall average amount of sleep shows only small changes for older groups, the range of individual differences in sleep amounts is clearly increased. Some people are sleeping much less and some are sleeping much more than is typical of a younger population. In the sleep-diary study noted above, while two-thirds of the 20-year-olds were averaging between 6 and 9 hours of sleep per night, two-thirds of the 60-year-olds were sleeping between 5 and 11 hours per night on the average.

Naps also show a consistent increase across time. While naps were seldom reported in the 20-year-old working population, nearly all the 60-year-olds reported napping and the group averaged nearly two naps per week.

An observational study of a group of very elderly men and women (average age 77) showed an extension of the trends we have noted. Two days of 24-hour observations were made. Night sleep was frequently interrupted. There was an average of 5.2 observable arousals. There were an average of nearly two nap periods per day (1.6) and nearly 10 percent of the sleep occurred during the day. The individual differences were large. One subject slept only 5 hours per 24 while four slept more than $9\frac{1}{2}$ hours. One subject had only two awakenings per night while half had five or more such awakenings. One subject took no naps during the two days; four had three or more naps per day. The males were significantly more variable than the females on most measures.

In spite of the age changes seen in this group of very elderly subjects and those cited earlier for the less aged, an important fact emerges. While the sleep process does show evidence of "fraying," more so in some persons than in others, it shows greater evidence of maintaining its integrity. In the substructure, REM and Stage 2 sleep are remarkably unchanged. Most of the sleep is still obtained in a long nocturnal period in spite of increased tendencies to interruption and the presence of naps. Amount of sleep is more markedly changed in variability than in total amount.

Implications of sleep and aging

Let me begin with three well-established facts about sleep and aging.

1. The patterns of sleep undergo natural and inherent changes associated with age.
2. There are wide individual differences in the pace and timing of these change processes.
3. Problems are more likely to occur as a result of our expectancies about sleep and our social needs than from sleep itself.

These statements hold particularly and dramatically true in the extremes of aging, i.e., before the ages of five and after the ages of fifty.

More specifically, we can expect dramatic changes to occur in the infant's patterns of sleep as a natural part of the maturation process. Sleep will change from being intermittent, dominant, and almost equally divided between night and day to becoming consolidated into long night periods and daytime naps by the end of the first year. The overall amount of sleep will have shown a gradual decline of several hours. This will all occur as a natural part of the child's heritage as a human. We can do our best to nurture and protect this process, but we can demand little of it in the way of satisfying our own desires or convenience. At worst we can do battle with it. Above all we can remember the wide range of individual differences. Sleep amounts in the newborn may differ by as much as 10 hours at birth and differences among young children of as much as 4 hours in sleep amount per 24 hours is not unusual. While half of all babies sleep through the night at the age of two months, half of them do not.

From the teens into the forties the major "natural" difference in sleep among persons will be in the amounts of sleep. There will be, of course, other variability within and between individuals but these will be imposed on a largely stable sleep structure.

The process of aging brings further developmental changes in sleep patterning. There are clear changes in the substructure, evidenced by diminishing amounts of deep sleep and increased awakenings and light sleep. These awakenings are reflected in the superstructure by awakenings and naps becoming more frequent. There are increases in individual differences within the same age group, resulting from the different rates of change in sleep characteristics as well as from changes in sleep itself.

Let us recognize that the great changes are primarily developmental ones. As such they are inherent, unlearned, and innate. There are at least three appropriate responses to such events. To recognize them, to be awed by them, and to provide the best environment possible in which they may unfold. The least appropriate response is to ignore their inherent nature and to believe that the infant or the aged person can perform as we wish rather than as they must.

5

The timing of sleep and waking

The tolerance by sleep of our other needs is one of our most valuable natural gifts. If, for example, we usually are awake for some 16 to 17 hours—say, from 7:00 A.M. to 11:00 P.M.—and we happen to need or want to stay awake longer, we can do so. How fortunate this is and what a different world it would be otherwise! Suppose we were "struck down" by sleep after those 16 to 17 hours while we were walking home from a late show. We would have to organize "sleep patrols" to come and gather up all those who had missed their time schedules from the sidewalks and benches and nooks and crannies where they had dropped into sleep and to deliver them to their beds. We could not get up early to go on trips or to study or go fishing. There would not be shift work and people who traveled across continents or oceans would be forever out of phase with the native residents. We would be helpless before our enemies and incapable of extending ourselves for transient pleasures or necessary responses. We would be trapped in the inexorable demands of a rigid set of boundaries in our life and much of its richness and resources would be lost. Dr. Seuss has given us a scene from such a world.

Fortunately, we can stay awake beyond our usual time of wakefulness, we can awaken from sleep after a limited period of time, and we can go to sleep at different times.

Sleep, however, is not insensitive to these impositions on its ways. In this chapter we shall see that the nature of sleep is modified in specific and increasingly predictable ways to each change in timing. We shall examine the effects of prolonging wakefulness, shortening sleep, and changing its onset times.

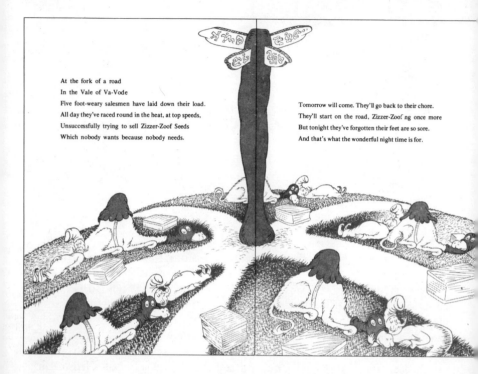

At the fork of a road
In the Vale of Va-Vode
Five foot-weary salesmen have laid down their load.
All day they've raced round in the heat, at top speeds,
Unsuccessfully trying to sell Zizzer-Zoof Seeds
Which nobody wants because nobody needs.

Tomorrow will come. They'll go back to their chore.
They'll start on the road, Zizzer-Zoofing once more
But tonight they've forgotten their feet are so sore.
And that's what the wonderful night time is for.

Variations in prior wakefulness

We vary the amount of time before we go to sleep for many reasons. We increase the time awake to study, to get somewhere, to continue enjoying ourselves as we look at the late shows on television, to finish a book, to be with friends, to pursue love. We also, though we more often overlook it, decrease the amount of time between sleep periods. We sleep late on weekends—say, until noon—and then try to go to bed at 11:00 P.M. after being awake for just eleven hours. We may decide to go to bed early because tomorrow is a "big day." We decide to take a nap some six hours after we have awakened.

These variations in prior wakefulness affect both the rate of going to sleep (sleep latency) and sleep length. Figure 5-1 shows the relationship between prior wakefulness and sleep latency.

This figure presents a simple set of facts about our sleep and waking behavior: the less time we are awake, the harder it is to get to sleep; and the longer we are awake, the stronger the tendency to go to sleep. Behaviorally, for example, it predicts what we have called "Sunday

FIG. 5-1   The relationship between the minutes taken to get to sleep (latency) and the amount of time of prior wakefulness.

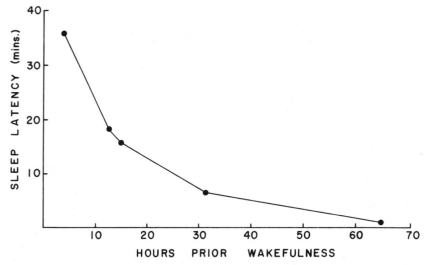

Source: Figure 2, p. 254 *Psychonomic Science*, vol. 24, no. 6, 1971.

night insomnia." If, as noted above, we sleep late on Sunday morning, say, until noon, and decide to go to bed early, at perhaps ten o'clock, because Monday is a big day, since we have been awake only ten hours there will be little tendency to go to sleep. We know less about the effect of an interjected nap, but the data does predict a reduced likelihood of going to sleep at night. On the other hand, it also predicts that if we have been awake for more than 20 hours we have an increased likelihood of going to sleep. If we think we are going to have trouble going to sleep on a particular night, we can increase the likelihood of sleeping by getting up particularly early the morning before or by staying up longer.

There is less data on the effect of prior wakefulness on sleep length, and the problem is more complicated. The complication comes from two directions. First, sleep has a built-in "self-destruct" mechanism. By this we mean that after a period of sleep there is a fortunate and natural tendency for us to stop sleeping. This tendency to wake up after a given time undoubtedly differs from person to person as to when it will occur; we have already seen that there are natural long and short sleepers. But for all of us, we don't just go on sleeping until something wakes us up. Rather we will begin to wake up ourselves after a given time period. Secondly, as we shall see in our look at the onset times of sleep, this tendency to wake up or be awake is tied to an overall rhythm of sleep and waking. The time to be asleep and the time to be awake have a natural rhythm in fairly regular sleepers. When we sleep out into the daytime hours we are trying to continue sleep in a "nonsleep" time and there will be a tendency to terminate sleep. There is, then, a time to sow and a time to sleep.

Perhaps, because of these complications, the little data that we have indicates that although there is probably a real relationship between prior wakefulness and sleep length it is by no means a strong or direct one. It is a common observation from sleep-deprivation experiments that, after prolonged wakefulness, individuals will sleep some 12 to 14 hours (although some will sleep only about 10 hours). Animal studies have shown that while sleep amount increases after deprivation, the amount of increase is not related to the amount of deprivation, for example, 24 versus 48 versus 72 hours of sleep loss. Further studies with rats, which are awake and asleep intermittently during the day and night, show no relationship between the immediately preceding amount of wakefulness and the immediately succeeding length of the sleep period. We know even less of the effect on sleep length of reducing the amount of prior wakefulness.

We clearly know less about the influence of prior wakefulness on sleep length than we should. My impression is that extended prior wakefulness will lengthen the sleep period within limits of the capacity to sleep and that short periods of prior wakefulness will limit sleep length (such as occurs in naps), but that the relationship is neither simple, strong, or direct.

The effects of prior wakefulness on the substructure of sleep have been studied in considerable detail. It has been found that the amount of time preceding a sleep period is directly but oppositely related to the amount of Stage 4 (deep sleep) and the amount of Stage 0 and Stage 1 appearing in sleep after sleep has begun (light sleep). If there are very few hours of wakefulness before one goes to sleep, there will be very little Stage 4 sleep and sleep will be interrupted or terminate early. As the length of wake time increases, up to about 20 hours, the amount of Stage 4 sleep steadily increases and the awakenings decrease. After about 20 hours of wakefulness, sleep will be as "deep" and "steady" as it can be unless the wakefulness is very prolonged, say, for 2 or 3 days. Under such circumstances Stage 4 sleep is very strong and there are no interruptions. In practical terms, if we try to get to sleep after we have been awake for less than about 16 hours, our sleep will be less deep and will be interrupted. An example would be our sleeping until noon and deciding to get a good night's sleep by going to bed early.

Prior wakefulness has a very small influence on Stage REM sleep.

Prolonged wakefulness will tend to reduce REM sleep but this is probably due to the strong dominance of Stage 4 sleep.

Variations in sleep length

Variations in the length of a sleep period result in sharply different "kinds" of sleep obtained in terms of the sleep stages.

The effects of variations in sleep length on the substructure of sleep are a direct result of the differential temporal distribution of sleep stages within sleep periods that we discussed in Chapter 3 and displayed in Figure 3-2. You will recall that Stage 4 occurs predominantly in the early part of the night and REM sleep increases in appearance in the later part of a full night's sleep. We have taken the data from this figure and calculated the effects on Stage 4 and REM of reducing sleep from eight hours to six hours or four hours, or increasing sleep to ten hours. We have also done our calculations for Stage 2, which is essentially equally present in each hour of sleep.

From these calculations, a reduction of sleep by 25 percent, from eight hours to six hours, results in a 36 percent reduction of REM sleep, a 25 percent reduction in Stage 2 (which appears essentially equal across hours), and only a 1 percent reduction in Stage 4 sleep. A 50 percent reduction in sleep, from eight to four hours, results in a differential "deprivation" or loss of 70 percent REM sleep, 50 percent Stage 2 sleep, and 2 percent Stage 4 sleep. Prolonging sleep by 25 percent, from eight to ten hours, enhances REM sleep and Stage 2 sleep with essentially no effect on Stage 4 sleep. Specifically, there is a 42 percent increase in REM sleep, 25 percent increase in Stage 2 sleep, and no increase in Stage 4 sleep.

In short, increases or decreases in sleep length have disproportionate effects on the REM stage but reductions to as little as four hours have only a limited effect on Stage 4 sleep.

Changes in sleep onset times

The time that we begin sleep is to a considerable extent under our own control. If we want to finish a book, or look at a late show, or pursue our pleasures, or are pushed by our problems, we simply go to bed later than usual. If the world has been too much with us, we may decide to go to bed early. We may, under the good fortune of schedules, be able to take a nap in the afternoon. In all these instances we change the usual time of going to sleep. If the changes in time are

significantly different from our "usual" time, or if they are very
erratic, they are likely to affect our sleep. However, even more
profound changes in sleep time are becoming a major aspect of many
people's lives today. This results from two conditions that have
emerged in our modern times: shift work and jet travel. In highly
industrialized settings, as many as one person in three is working on
shift or work schedules other than the standard work period from 8 to
5, and the sleep of such persons is displaced within this new schedule.
Millions of passengers per year travel on long jet flights across multiple
time zones, which "displaces" their sleep periods. A person flying from
New York to Paris, for example, must "move" his sleep period forward
by six hours to have his sleep in line with the Parisian sleep/waking
world.

We can best understand the problems involved by citing four facts
that have emerged from recent experimental studies of sleep and
performance under shift-work conditions and jet displacements.

1. The timing of the sleep stages within sleep is radically altered.
Earlier we showed how a period of sleep "transferred" from an 11:00
P.M. to 8:00 A.M. onset time had an altered pattern (Figure 3-3). Figure
5-2 shows what happens to the appearance of REM sleep and Stage 4
sleep across the 24 hours. This figure gives the amount of these stages
of sleep in the first two hours of sleep at varying points during the day
and night. Clearly REM sleep "crowds" into the sleep period early in

FIG. 5-2   The percentage of time occupied by Stage 4 and Stage REM in two-hour
sleep periods beginning at different times during the day.

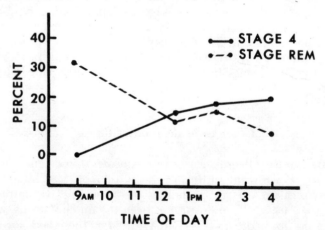

Source: Figure 1, p. 32 of *Aspects of Human Efficiency,* ed. W. P. Colquhoun (London: The
English Universities Press, Ltd., 1972).

day sleep and diminishes in this tendency toward the "usual" sleep time. There is a converse effect relative to Stage 4. In short, there is clear evidence that our sleep during the day is different from our regular sleep.

2. Sleep occurring during the usual waking time (day sleep) is more broken (a sharp increase in number of arousals and Stage 1) and is often terminated early (the length of the sleep period is reduced).

3. Performance during the usual sleep period sharply deteriorates. When the individual tries to perform tasks from about midnight to 8:00 A.M., those tasks that are sensitive to sleep loss show reduced efficiency during this time even when no sleep deprivation is present; errors increase and experimenter-paced tasks, particularly of the long-term and low-motivation type, show decrements.

4. When the new schedule is maintained for a period of time, the sleep patterns reorganize themselves into their original form and performance improves during the original sleep period. The rate of adaptation varies according to the functions measured and varies among individuals; some functions show rapid adaptations while others may show shift effects over several weeks.

These four facts add up to one general conclusion: sleep and waking take place within a complex set of biological rhythms. In its stable form sleep shows strong and certain peaks and troughs of modulated functions. When the timing of this rhythm is modified, the original rhythms persist. The resultant conflicts between the new demands and the old rhythm are evident and a new rhythm must be developed. Stated otherwise, it may be said that there is a natural time to sleep and a time to be active which the body "knows" and utilizes: under a new schedule it adapts its rhythm to that new schedule.

Occasional variations of limited displacements are likely to have little effect on the basic rhythm of sleep and waking. However, some effects of the variant rhythms on sleep and performance are likely to be present. If a person "works" until, say, 4:00 A.M., past his or her usual 11:00 P.M. bedtime, this will be "uphill" since the tendencies to go to sleep because it is "sleep time" will be there. These will be compounded by a prolonged time of prior wakefulness. Further, efficiency of performance is likely to be reduced since performance is occurring in the sleep trough. When sleep does occur, REM is likely to have a shortened latency and appear early. If sleep then continues on into the waking period, sleep may be broken and terminate early.

Variations in sleep-onset times across short time bands such as four hours may have a more subtle but disturbing effect. Since this is a rhythm, a stable time system is desirable. If sleep occurs on one night at 2:00 A.M., and the next night at 10:00 P.M., and on the third night

the individual decides to go to sleep at midnight, in oversimplified
terms the sleep system is likely to be saying, "What's going on up
there? One night I'm supposed to be asleep at this time and the next
night I'm supposed to be awake. Which is it tonight?" Given no stable
cues for onset—no rhythmic help in determining whether sleep should
occur or not occur—the response is likely to be unstable. In a study
conducted several years ago, the strongest predictor of "I go to sleep
easily" was "I go to sleep at a regular hour." Of course, regularity may
correlate with many other things that increase the likelihood of
untroubled sleep onset, but it is not unreasonable to believe that the
regularity, in and of itself, is a strong aid to an easy sleep onset.

Beyond, however, our self-imposed variation in time of sleep, the
presence of shift work in our industrialized society poses one of the
major problems of sleep. Industrial surveys emphasize the magnitude,
the size, and the consequences of this problem. As early as 1951 it was
reported that in English industries employing 10 or more persons,
more than $2\frac{1}{4}$ million workers were on shifts. Further, the Ministry of
Labor in 1965 reported a 50 percent rise in shift work over the
preceding decade. Ten years ago in Holland almost one-fourth of
Dutch workers were on shift schedules. In America the amount of shift
work varies widely by locale, but the percentages are remarkably high.
In 1961 the Bureau of Labor Statistics reported the following figures
for the percentage of shift workers in a number of cities: Detroit—33
percent, St. Louis—25 percent, Seattle—24 percent, New York—13
percent. The above figures reflect primarily statistics within industrial
programs. In addition there is a broad spectrum of workers in
transportation, health care, entertainment, law enforcement, sanita-
tion, and communications who work on varied shifts. There is an
increasing extension of service facilities in response to the presence of
the shift worker: clerks in drugstores, food stores, and the like. To all
these numbers must be added the families of shift workers, who in
many ways also feel the impact of shift work.

There is not likely to be an abatement of this increasingly 24-hour
world. The forces behind this phenomenon—the availability of 24
hours of light and heat, the high cost of production units that must be
continuously used to be economical, the increased number of continu-
ous-processing plants, competitive pressure—are more likely to increase than decrease.

Industrial survey studies have repeatedly attested to problems
associated with shift work that are congruent with the facts we have
outlined above. Over one-half of shift workers in a study from
Germany had complaints about their sleep, specifying both insufficient sleep and inferior quality during the day. A careful review of

the industrial studies by one source stated that all "worker-oriented" studies to date had found difficulties in sleep as a frequent source of complaint. Two studies singled out sleep as *the* central problem for shift workers. One study found that 83 percent of the men sampled felt "most tired" in the night shift, with only 4 percent making such a statement about their day-shift work.

In addition to sleep problems, from 25 to 50 percent of night-shift workers complained about lack of appetite and digestion-elimination difficulties. Some researchers have found evidence of more severe intestinal disorders. There has been substantial evidence of increased errors and diminished production during the night shift.

There is a simple biological solution to the problems of shift work, but unfortunately it is not likely to be utilizable for some time. We are in the position of the old farmer whose son, recently returned from agricultural college, began telling him how to farm better. "Son," he said, "I already know how to farm twice as good as I'm able to."

The solution is, of course, permanent shifts, since sleep/waking rhythms do adapt over time and become stably reorganized in a new time period. In such regimes, day becomes the "natural" sleep time and night becomes the "natural" work time. The problem, however, lies in the worker's social recreation and family life remaining organized to the "daytime" world. The shift worker prefers to be out of biological phase occasionally rather than out of social phase chronically. As a result of these social pressures, industrial shifts, rather than being permanent, are more typically swiftly rotating shifts. On the commonly used Metropolitan Shift the worker moves across three shifts in two-day intervals. In another common model the worker takes the night shift for a block of one week once every month.

In general, industry has responded to these problems by incentive pay, compensatory time, and increased quality control and safety standards for the "off" shifts. These compensate for some of the social problems involved but are not likely to reduce the inherent biological problem. Perhaps a more "around-the-clock" world will improve the social consequences of shift work. Certainly considerable further analyses of shift times are called for. Minimally, the worker must become sensitive to the consequences of shifts and attempt to develop helpful strategies of his own.

The "jet lag" problem, fortunately for most of us, tends to be an infrequent affair and then associated with vacations rather than work requirements. However, for airline personnel, businessmen, military, and governmental officials jet travel poses much the same problem as that posed for the shift worker: the necessity to adapt to a new time schedule for sleep and waking. Note the problems of a typical night flight from New York to London: departure at 10:00 P.M. New York time; six hours of flight; arrival at 10:00 A.M. London time (4:00 A.M. New York time). One now has the poor choice of going to bed on arrival in London, since it is one's old biorhythm time for sleep, or gritting one's teeth, rubbing one's eyes and proceeding through the day. Taking the latter course, after an early dinner one could retire at 9:00 P.M. London time, which is 3:00 P.M. New York time. Fortunately, one is probably so exhausted under this choice that sleep even in the daytime is likely to occur easily. Unfortunately, because one has gone to bed so early, awakening is likely to occur after about nine hours—when it will be only 6:00 A.M. London time. However, this is also midnight New York time and one must now begin to function through one's usual sleep time for some six to eight hours.

There have been arguments in the literature regarding the relative ease of east to west flights (moving time forward) versus west to east flights (moving time backward). A prominent factor that must be taken into account is the arrival time in the new environment. For example, if the traveler departs New York at 10:00 A.M. rather than 10:00 P.M., he arrives in London in the evening, at about 10:00 P.M. London time, and the surround encourages the beginning of his new cycle. A late dinner and bedding down about midnight will have him going to sleep early on New York time (about 6:00 P.M.) but at least he has begun to be in step with London time. One can work out a very good or very poor schedule of flights from west to east relative to arrival time.

A second factor that seems likely to have an influence, particularly for airline personnel, would be whether they are returning to "home base" or their "home rhythm" rather than to a new one, regardless of whether it was an east-to-west or a west-to-east flight.

While the biorhythm problems are fundamentally the same, there are two real differences between the jet-lag situation and the shift-work situation. First, the time shift associated with the jet-lag problem is typically preceded by the intensive activity of travel itself. This is particularly true for the airline personnel. Secondly, the surround after a jet flight is in "support" of the new shifted rhythm; that is, the new "night" sleep will in fact occur at night, whereas the shift worker is actually sleeping during the day. This support by the physical conditions is certainly likely to facilitate adaptation in the long run to the new pattern resulting from jet flights. It must at the same time, however, be recognized as a force that may be "pushing" the new behavior. The person may be falsely assured by the new environment that he can proceed without taking into account the fact that this is an entirely new rhythm. Certainly travelers need to recognize the impositions on their systems resulting from time displacements. Seasoned airline personnel and diplomats follow one of two strategies. Either they "ease" into the situation, as in our first example above, by sleeping for at least several hours on arrival; or, if the trip is a brief one, that is, the turn around to home is short, they maintain home time as closely as the situation permits—for example, by holding meetings in the evenings, which in an east-west flight is "daytime" for them.

Interactions

As noted in an earlier chapter, these variations in time, which are, in fact, variations in the superstructure of sleep—prior wakefulness, length, and onset time—may occur independently but in fact are typically interactive and the effects compounded. This is best seen at the onset of a worker going on a midnight shift. He may work through his usual sleep time, say, 11:00 P.M. until 8:00 A.M., and then go to bed. If he were to get up at 8:00 A.M. before his shift his prior wakefulness would be 24 hours, his onset time shifted by 9 hours, and his sleep length would be either increased by the prolonged prior wakefulness or decreased because of "day sleep." He could instead try taking a long nap from 4:00 P.M. to 8:00 P.M. before the shift. In this schedule he would have "double-shifted" his onset times (4:00 P.M. and 8:00 P.M.), his prior wakefulness times (8 hours and 12 hours), and his sleep length (4 hours and perhaps 6 hours).

Implications

There are a few important ways that sleep within a 24-hour period may in fact be modified: sleep may be held off or begun early (prior wakefulness varied), sleep length may be reduced or extended, sleep onset time may be shifted, or all these factors may be modified together. Sleep itself is systematically affected by each of these changes. Prior-wakefulness time increases or decreases the tendency to go to sleep and affects the structure of sleep by particularly increasing or decreasing the amount of deep sleep. Reduction in sleep length results in a differential deprivation of REM sleep and has some effect on subsequent sleep length. Changes in onset time disrupt the rhythm of sleep and affect performance.

These are all "natural" changes that we may impose voluntarily on our sleep—a late show, an early fishing trip, an intensive demand on our time—or are increasingly imposed by our contemporary society in the form of shift work or jet travel.

The understandable, scientifically "law-abiding" character of these variations in timing makes it increasingly possible to accurately predict the consequences of what happens when, voluntarily or involuntarily, the change in sleep/waking patterns occurs.

These findings emphasize the systematic nature of sleep. It is at once a sensitive system as it responds to variations in its basic format and a self-protective system as it attempts to maintain its integrity in the face of imposed variations in its form.

6

Conditions prior to and during sleep

Sleep is inevitably preceded by what we do each day, what we think about, how we feel, and what happens to us. Where we sleep is surrounded by physical space and particular conditions. This chapter focuses on these precursors of sleep and the surround during sleep.

These variables, the immediate precursors and the surround, may be classified as "state" variables. These variables are transient, ahistorical, and situational. Typical are the amount of work we do from day to day or noise levels while we sleep. Their effects on sleep would be immediate and the resultant changes in the sleep process would be in direct response to these conditions. Sleep may serve to compensate for our being particularly tired or having learned a great deal, or it may be disrupted or disturbed by such conditions. However, as the "state" changes, sleep would return to its natural "base."

The precursors of sleep

We will first concern ourselves with the immediate precursors of sleep. In particular we will focus on variations that occur in our daytime activities preceding a particular sleep period. Even confining ourselves to this narrow range of time leaves a vast variety of potential variables. The world preceding sleep is as infinitely varied as the world itself and our reactions to it. We may laugh, dance, be idle or busy, run or walk, be sad or happy, learn much or little, be frightened or simply drift awash in our routines. These events stretch across time from our awakening to our going to bed. Any or all of these happenings and responses to them may or may not affect the sleep that follows.

To simplify things let us first consider the effects of more or less amounts of our routine behavior before we turn to the more extreme conditions of threats to or extensions of behavior patterns. We will first ask what are the effects on sleep of our ordinary day-to-day activities . . . eating somewhat more or less, being more or less energetic or sociable, reading or learning more, getting a little angrier or sadder, or being a little more fulfilled than usual.

Studies of these day-to-day variations are quite sparse but the few that have been conducted are very informative. There are several reasons for this lack of data. Undoubtedly one important factor is the recency of our research efforts, which has resulted in our working on more obvious and pressing problems. Another, certainly, relates to the difficulties in the measurement, coding, and control of day-to-day kinds of variables. It is very difficult to measure and define, much less control, how "happy" or "interested" a person was during a particular day. It is also likely that some of the lack of data stems from the generally discouraging lack of as yet observable effect of such variables. Experimenters, being very human, prefer to work on problems that yield significant results.

We can illustrate these problems by describing an experiment we conducted in our laboratory recently. Forty volunteers reported to our laboratory at their usual bedtime in groups of four.

An elaborate procedure was developed to obtain a description of their daily activities. For each person each half hour of the day was reviewed and recorded. In addition, a checklist of "more than usual—less than usual" ratings of some 15 items was used as a probe and to rate each half hour: "Were you more or less than usually involved in learning new material?" "More or less involved in talking to others?" etc. An extensive battery of mood scales was administered: "happy-sad," "bored-interested," "calm-excited," etc., were some of the categories included. All of this data was scaled and, in turn, related to the variables of sleep such as latency of onset, length, stages, and even "good" or "poor" sleep evaluations after sleep.

The relationships obtained were not impressive. We compared 22 daytime "event" or "state" measures against 12 sleep measures. The strongest relationships barely exceeded chance and there were very few of these.

This study may never see the light of literature along with an unknown but probably large number of studies that have attempted to relate the effects of studying versus nonstudying, good moods versus bad moods, high attention levels versus low attention levels, etc., to sleep. In my own files there are a number of such studies moldering amid a mass of negative results.

There are good and poor reasons for such results not being published. Journals are already overcrowded with positive relationships. Experimenters don't like to report on their failures. The best reason, however, is that the lack of obtained relationships may not be due to the absence of relationship, but perhaps results from poor experiments. The measures used may not have reflected the underlying effect. Had we measured the real "moods"? The effective variables may have been missed by the net that was cast. Perhaps feelings of "sexiness" were affecting sleep stages and we didn't measure this feeling. It is possible that the variables didn't vary enough in most of the subjects and that this obscured the effect in the few subjects in which the effect was present. We may not have measured the aspects of sleep that were affected. If the experiment was inadequate, to report no relationship is not to report information but misinformation.

In the case of the precursors of sleep we are fortunate in having a set of experiments that suggest very strongly a real lack of effect rather than experimental error. In these experiments a certainly measurable, easily controllable, and very logically related precursor has been carefully studied: the amount of physical energy or exercise taken prior to sleep.

The amount of exercise in such studies is easily and carefully controlled, most often by using exercise bicycles geared to various work loads. The first study did indeed find an effect, although an unexpected one. Heavy exercise was introduced in the evening before the sleep period. Instead of increasing deep sleep, exercise in fact decreased deep sleep. Reasoning that the results were probably not due to the exercise but to a generalized activation of the system intruding into sleep, another study was done. This subsequent study placed the exercise in the daytime, with the resulting marginal but significant effect of increasing deep sleep with little or no effect on the other stages.

In light of these results a number of laboratories, including ours, attempted to use exercise as an experimental variable that would purposefully modify deep sleep. There was typically no effect. There was also the puzzling fact that no exercise or limited energy expenditure such as is seen in bed-rest conditions showed no effect. More recently a very careful exercise study performed in Canada failed to find any effect on sleep. The weight of evidence is rather clear. Exercise has little or no effect on sleep patterns.

We would argue that these experiments strongly support the notion that day-to-day variations within limits have little effect on the sleep "package." Here is a variable which, among the many variations possible, could be expected to have an effect but which careful study does not find to be a significant factor.

There are no studies that I know of which deny this conclusion, and, of course, there is no way of fully confirming a "non"-effect. There is, however, considerable indirect data to support this position of a limited effect on sleep. A number of studies have been conducted to determine the effect of previous stimulation on dream content. Vivid and stressful movies were shown and the dream recall compared to that following the showing of nonstressful movies. Often dream content or vividness was changed but the sleep measures showed essentially no changes. The most compelling findings have been those indicating the lack of difference in sleep patterns among individuals who live very different lives. As we shall see, the sleep patterns of institutionalized schizophrenics differ little or none from those of "normals." These individuals—living in an institutionalized, almost desocialized, autistic world, and acting in bizarre ways—sleep the sleep of normals, unaffected by the nature of their day-to-day behavior. The same may be said for mental retardates, whose learning or reading capacity is very different from your world and mine. Their sleep shows little or no differences from ours.

Of particular interest is the remarkably consistent lack of difference between the sleep of males and females. Before the recent "women's liberation" wars there were quite different day-to-day differences between males and females in physical activities and varying attitudinal, situational, and emotional aspects of life. Many still exist, including a variety of physiological differences. Yet all the studies indicate that these day-to-day ways of being have little effect on differences in sleep characteristics.

This lack of differences makes biological sense. Sleep is an organized system that is set to perform a repeated function. If it required continual readjustments to meet each mood change or minor variations in the way we feel or act, the demands would be excessive. We may use an analogy here. Sleep as a system can be considered somewhat similar to digestion. Fortunately for us, digestion pursues its hidden and complex ways, performs its ordained job, reasonably independent of our voluntary control or our daily peccadilloes. If it were required to work differently as we routinely vary our day, it would not be as effective a system.

We are not, of course, saying that sleep or digestion is totally unaffected by what the world does to us or what we do within that world. Recall that we have been talking about relatively mild variations of our routine lives. There are effects of more extreme variations—peaks and troughs that are essentially qualitative changes or events in our lives. A critical decision to be made, an all-important examination, a blossoming love affair—aspects of life that threaten or extend our well-being beyond its usual boundaries—what of their effect on sleep?

Again the dimensions are manifold and the data almost completely nonexistent. However, the lack of data in this instance stems not from a probable lack of effect but rather from problems of experimental conditions. These conditions cannot be effectively created in the laboratory and, when they do exist, the opportunity or even the propriety of studying them is problematic. One simply doesn't approach someone in deep trouble or in a peak experience and say, "Pardon me, would you now come into my laboratory and show me your sleep?"

We would certainly argue that these precursors of sleep—states of high elation, depression, or conflict—will affect sleep. Our reasoning is based on two simple but reasonable assumptions for which there is considerable supportive data.

For one thing, the need to maintain wakefulness and the need for sleep are independent and negatively interactive. When one is significantly elevated it may override or interfere with the other.

Under strong motivation, to remain awake is the natural response whether it is to defend or extend oneself. Under such circumstances sleep is often suppressed voluntarily: "I can't go to sleep for I must keep studying to pass the examination"; "I don't want to go to sleep, I'm enjoying this too much."

However, from habit, thoughts about tomorrow's work, the press of sleep itself, we often try to sleep while still under the pressure of strong motivations created by our daily existence. Under these circumstances sleep is likely to be affected. These conscious and unconscious needs carry with them tendencies to remain awake and their degree will determine the extent to which sleep is disturbed. As we continue to respond to these needs, we will be "situational" insomniacs. Wakefulness has penetrated and persevered into the sleep period.

The most obvious effect is on sleep onset. So long as we keep reacting to the high-motive state we have brought to the sleep period we will remain awake. The two masters cannot be served at the same time. Our second assumption, therefore, is that as long as we are, consciously or unconsciously, rehearsing or reliving "the things that we have done and left undone"—behaving in relation to them—sleep will have small room for occurrence. Only gradually, from a pressure of sleep need or a fading of the other pressures via distraction or resignation, will sleep finally take its place.

Even after sleep has begun, strong needs may assert their place. Although there have been few systematic studies of sleep under stress or high-motive conditions, we are becoming very familiar with the patterns of "stressed" sleep in our studies of psychopathology and insomnias (Chapters 9 and 11). The pattern of individuals under "chronic" stress is one of many awakenings, frequent sleep stage changes, and early awakenings. Within sleep, light sleep (Stage 1) markedly increases and deep sleep (Stages 3 and 4) show drastic decreases.

The effects of the sleep surroundings

Although somewhat more restricted than our waking world, the surround of sleep is varied and complex. This can be seen in the Dr. Seuss illustration of the Zwieback Motel. We sleep on mountains and

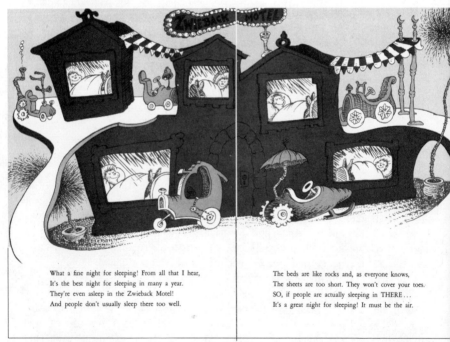

What a fine night for sleeping! From all that I hear,
It's the best night for sleeping in many a year.
They're even asleep in the Zwieback Motel!
And people don't usually sleep there too well.

The beds are like rocks and, as everyone knows,
The sheets are too short. They won't cover your toes.
SO, if people are actually sleeping in THERE . . .
It's a great night for sleeping! It must be the air.

in valleys, in familiar home settings and motels, alone and together. The physical elements have great range. It may be hot or cold. There may be almost no sound or we may be near a bustling airport. The bed may be soft or hard. We may sleep naked or in elaborate night attire. We import into these scenes the motives and residues of the day that we discussed above and there are those evoked by the sleep situation itself. How does this cacophony affect sleep?

An important aspect of sleep needs emphasis at this point. Sleep is a highly adaptive process. It is, at once, sensitive to its surround and is self-protective as a continuing process. When we go to sleep we do not become completely independent of our surround and unloosen totally our continuing relation to what is going on. A most commonly held belief—that mothers may awaken to the faint whimper of their child after having slept through immediately preceding rumbles of trucks, cracks of thunder, or blasts of low-flying jet aircraft—is true. This illustration points up the twofold adaptive nature of sleep. The mother *was* awakened by the child but *not* awakened by the "irrelevant" or "nonsensitized" sounds. In considering, then, the effect of the surround we must never simply talk about the physical event itself but keep in mind the "meaning" of the event as it evokes a response or permits the response to be ignored.

We can best explore the effects of the surround on sleep by reviewing what we know about the relationship between sleep and a particular, obvious, and important surround variable that has had rather extensive exploration—the effect of noise on sleep. Like exercise, in the previous section, this is an easily controlled and obviously highly relevant variable.

A look at the data from studies of this factor emphasizes the complexity of making generalizations about surround conditions. Here are some of the findings:

1. The sleep stage that a person is in makes a difference. In response to a standard signal, there is essentially a direct, negative relationship between the intensity of the signal required to obtain a response and sleep stages 1, 2, 3, and 4 in that order. Responses from Stage 1 require less stimulation than from Stage 4.

2. At any given sleep stage there is a relationship between the intensity of the signal and the probability of a response. Simply stated, low intensities may not wake a person up but loud noises will.

3. The age of the subject is an important factor. Younger subjects are less responsive than older subjects.

4. The level of arousal in sleep is an issue in deciding the effect of a stimulus. EEG arousal may occur without behavioral arousal.

A recent paper emphasizes points 3 and 4. Three groups were tested on their response to simulated sonic booms and jet flyovers: children from 5 to 8; middle-aged subjects from 41 to 57; older subjects from 65 to 79. None of the children woke up, while 12 and 35 percent of the middle-aged and older subjects woke up. On EEG criteria, a significant change in the EEG with or without arousal, 12 percent of the children responded while 36 and 60 percent of the middle-aged and older subjects responded on the signs.

5. The "relevance" of the signal has an important influence. We are more sensitive to "meaningful" sounds than neutral ones. Animal studies show them to be highly responsive to very low-level, "threatening" natural sounds when compared with neutral tones. We can "condition" a person to be extrasensitive to a tone paired with shock. An example of this complex influence is seen in studies in which one particular sound meant that the subject must wake up to avoid a shock while other sounds were simply noises. In studies of sounds alone, the response was more sensitive (required lower stimulation) in Stages 1 through 4 than in REM sleep. During REM sleep the subjects were even less sensitive to the neutral tone than when in Stage 4. However, the subjects showed equal sensitivity to relevant or shock-warning tones during REM as in Stage 2 sleep.

6. The question of "adaptation" is complex and controversial ("controversial" perhaps because it is complex). We know from experience that we can sleep within repeated and familiar noisy conditions. But if we mean by "adaptation" physiologically becoming unresponsive to a repeated stimulus, then the weight of the data indicates that adaptation is limited. With repetition after repetition of, for example, sonic booms, subjects continue to respond physiologically (EEG, etc.). However, from our discussion of relevance we know that subjects show limited responses to "nonadaptive" stimuli. The latter fact suggests that "motivation" or "knowledge" interacts with the physical stimulus and, although the person continues to be physiologically sensitive, the repeated repetition of a sound brings a "motivational" or "knowledge" desensitization of the response to that stimulation—in other words, no awakening or behavior to noise.

7. The pattern of the sounds is a similarly complex problem. Continuing or steady noises have little effect on sleep. However, sharp changes in level or patterns of sound do have effects on sleep. Significantly, however, changes in the environment are signals about the "meaning" of the environment and we are thrown back to the issue of relevance. An excellent illustration of this is seen in the "miller's response" discussed in the early 1870s. In attempting to understand the effects of noise, the paradox of the miller who ground wheat by use of a waterwheel in a stream was noted. When this continuous squeaking and rumbling would stop, the miller would immediately awaken to the silence!

8. The degree of disruption of sleep will be dependent upon the nature of the response signaled and the nature of the environmental

requirements. This relates to item 4 above. Sleep has a "built-in" tendency to continue. An EEG arousal or even a brief behavioral awakening will most likely be followed by continued sleep. Indeed, the particular sleep stage that the person is in at the signal time has the highest probability of continuing. As a result of this, single or intermittent arousals that require no "nonsleep" action by the individual are likely to have minimal effects on the total sleep of the person. A loud, sudden sound may completely awaken a person for a few seconds or a minute but this will be followed by sleep and probably yield no recall in the morning. The total effect would be to "change" sleep by 1/480th in an eight-hour sleep period. On the other hand a relevant signal (the baby crying, a possible intruder), or a high-response demand (Fire!) or a fragile sleep pattern associated with age may finish sleep for the night or, at least, for a significant period of time.

What, then, must we take into account in talking of sleep as it is affected by noise? At least the seven factors outlined above must be considered. When in sleep does the sound occur? How loud is the sound? How old is the subject? What response is present? What does the sound signal? How often has the sound occurred? What is the pattern of change in the sound? Only by having the answers to these questions, at least, can we answer questions about the sound surround on sleep. Given these answers we can begin to answer specifics: Can we be affected by airplanes taking off? Can I hear a burglar? How noisy can an air conditioner be?

We can draw some general conclusions. If sleep occurs within some reasonable ranges of familiar noises it proceeds to fulfill itself within its "buffer" of reduced sensitivity. It continues, however, to be responsive to and, in this sense, disrupted by extremes of noise and highly relevant signals, and the degree of disruption will be dependent upon the response required.

What about all of the other physical conditions that surround sleep and may vary widely? We are in essentially the same position here that we were in regarding the precursors, and probably for the same general reasons. The studies are not numerous—probably because, within limited ranges of conditions, the effects are quite limited.

Restricting ourselves to a limited range of physical variations—for want of a better term, "routine" variations—it is likely that the effects on sleep are quite limited. Somewhat more heat or cold, somewhat more light or less, a somewhat different bed, a set of different smells: none of these should make very much difference in sleep. Whatever the effects, they would also be predictable along the principles underlying the findings regarding sound: stimulus magnitude, sleep stages, subject age, frequency of stimulation, pattern of stimulation and, above all, the relevance or meaning of the stimulations.

Our reasoning about the limited effect is the same as that given for the effect of the precursors. The system, to be most effective, should be (and is) stable in relation to essentially irrelevant input.

An excellent example of the stability of this system and its generally limited response to the sleep surround is found in studies of the "first night" effect in laboratories. In laboratory recordings over many nights we have consistently found that people do indeed show patterns of slightly disturbed sleep in the first night in the laboratory. There are more awakenings, lighter sleep, more stage changes, less Stage 4, and often a slight decrease in REM sleep. However, even despite the wires hanging from their heads and the fact of sleeping in a strangely silent room with someone watching all night, the subjects' responses are typically quite mild. Most important, sleep on the second night has "adapted." It will be little different, after the first night, when measured night after night. The very strange surround has had a limited effect restricted to one night!

We have discussed the role of the "imported" thoughts and motives that enter into the sleep surround in relation to the precursors. They are incompatible with sleep. If they are strong enough to elicit continuing defensive or extensive responses they will affect sleep. If they prevent the onset of sleep they are potential intruders into the ongoing sleep.

Again we must emphasize that we are not saying that the surround has no effect on sleep. Rather, we would point up the adaptive nature of sleep in relation to the surround. On the one hand sleep appears capable of "dampening" and "filtering" out the surround, and as a result minor and routine variations in the environment have a limited effect on sleep. On the other hand, it is by no means flatly impervious to the surround; it permits awakening to significant changes in the surround when these are defined by either the magnitude or significance of the signals present.

Implications

Each of our lives and each of our days is constituted of constantly and widely varying conditions and behaviors. These result in complex "states" of being. The data indicates that, within broad ranges, sleep is generally unaffected by our daily doings. It appears to be an organized system that runs its routine course night after night and finds no reasons to do more or less in the face of our being more or less what we were yesterday, but rather performs its duty in its own basic ways. This is a most valuable character of sleep, since it requires no continual readjustment or compensation for our being who we are.

However, sleep can be and is affected by events in time. When these events and behaviors create "states" that bring with them continuing thoughts and motives for action, these will be incompatible with sleep. When the day has evoked strong needs to defend or extend ourselves they will certainly be incompatible with sleep. This, too, is as it should be since it permits us to respond to extraordinary pressures on us and to matters of extended concern.

Once sleep has begun it shows its adaptive nature. As with the precursors of sleep, there is an inherent capacity to "dampen" or ignore changes in the environment that are limited, routine, or irrelevant. If the sleep surround remains pretty much as we expect it to be or have come to know it, sleep will continue in its routine ways. At the same time it remains capable of yielding to significant changes of a demanding environment. Signals of tigers—real or imagined— can penetrate the sleep envelope.

7

Individual differences in sleep

In the last chapter we considered the influence on sleep of varying "states" arising from day-to-day activities or the sleep environment. Changes in the world around us or in our behavior result in "states": we work hard and we are "tired"; we don't eat and we are "hungry"; we hear a sound and become "alert." In this chapter, however, we are concerned with "traits." These are characteristics of ourselves that remain essentially the same across time and situations. They form consistent differences among individuals. The most obvious of these differences are physical. We are short or tall, fat or thin, have large ears or small. Some traits are less heavily determined biologically and more directly affect our behavior. These are influenced to varying degrees by our environments. We are more or less intelligent, more or less agile or skillful, more or less musically endowed. And there are the complicated "personality" traits. These are heavily influenced by our environment in their development. We are shy or aggressive, optimistic or pessimistic, hostile or friendly, anxious or serene.

This division between state and trait variables is oversimplified since state and trait variables may interact. A person may be in a "state of anxiety" due to a threatening circumstance; a series of threatening circumstances or "states" may result in the development of a "trait" of anxiety; a "trait" of anxiety may create a "state" of anxiety in a perfectly nonthreatening circumstance. Further, the idea of a "trait" smacks of a person "having" it or not. In fact, traits exist only in degrees and furthermore tend to be mixed within each person. A person may be an introvert in the midst of "strangers," but an "extrovert" with close friends. Nevertheless, consistent differences do exist among people and these, when quite strong in degree, can make considerable differences in behavior.

In relation to sleep we must ask two questions: Are there sleep traits and if so are they related to other differences? (Certainly the illustration of the Biffer-Baum by Dr. Seuss suggests that there are such traits at least across species.) Do consistent individual differences or trait differences among people influence sleep?

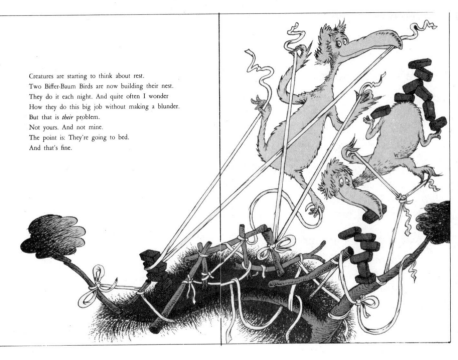

Creatures are starting to think about rest.
Two Biffer-Baum Birds are now building their nest.
They do it each night. And quite often I wonder
How they do this big job without making a blunder.
But that is *their* problem.
Not yours. And not mine.
The point is: They're going to bed.
And that's fine.

Sleep traits

While the earlier chapters on the effects of age and time variations recognized individual differences in sleep, or sleep traits, our emphasis was on the "average" effects of these variations. Stage 4, for example decreased with age but increased with amount of prior wakefulness; REM sleep stayed constant with age beyond the early teens and was shifted in time by changing the sleep onset. However, these were average effects or effects on groups. Within a given condition there was a wide range of individual differences. Although the average sleep length decreased by one-half from birth to young adulthood, there were individuals sleeping a great deal more or less than that average at any given age. Although the Stage 4 sleep was markedly diminished in an older group, some individuals had essentially none and others a substantial amount. Our emphasis at this point is on these differences among individuals. Are they consistent differences or traits being shown by individuals?

The most obvious difference among individuals in their sleep is a difference in the amount of sleep needed. Let us recall some of these differences that we have already noted. Among the newborn the amount of sleep varies from 22 hours to $10\frac{1}{2}$ in each 24-hour period. In the study of the first six months of the sleep of 19 infants, one child averaged 12 hours per night while another averaged 16 hours per night. In the group of 40 students who kept sleep logs for two weeks, one student averaged 6 hours while another averaged 10 hours per night.

Large samples confirm this wide range. From self-reports of typical sleep in the previous year by over 4,000 entering students at the University of Florida, 7 percent reported less than $6\frac{1}{2}$ hours of sleep per night and 3 percent more than $9\frac{1}{2}$ hours per night. These self-reported differences are affirmed by the more laborious sleep diary procedures. Two hundred and forty persons between the ages of 20 and 70 kept a diary of their sleep for eight weeks. Twenty percent slept less than 7 hours per night and 5 percent slept more than 9 hours per night.

Striking evidence of differences in sleep length is seen in two laboratory studies of short sleepers. Two healthy and effectively functioning males between 30 and 40 years of age were found to sleep consistently less than three hours per night. An elderly 70-year-old woman slept approximately one hour per night.

To be considered traits these differences must be consistent across time. Unfortunately, hard data is somewhat limited on this question. But the self-reports are statements about "usual" or consistent sleep patterns, and interviews have affirmed the general ability of people to report on their sleep lengths, particularly in the extremes. Sleep-log data has shown substantial consistencies from week to week. Bolstered by this and common sense we can accept the fact that there is a trait of natural and substantial differences in sleep length.

The data on sleep traits *within* sleep is substantial and surprising. There have been many measurements of sleep stages across a number of nights. Considering "normal" subjects, that is, individuals without significant complaints or unusual sleep habits or lengths, several consistent findings emerge. The amount of deep sleep (Stage 4) and light sleep (Stage 1) remains highly consistent from night to night. These stages show evidence of being traits. On the other hand, the amount of REM sleep and the latency of sleep onset vary from night to night and act more like state variables.

There are other characteristics of sleep that show tendencies of both consistency and inconsistency. Indeed, inconsistency itself may be paradoxically consistent. Sleep placement relative to onset and arousal times may be very regular (consistent), or somewhat regular, or consistently inconsistent. Another example is that there are consistently high, low, and occasional dream recallers.

We can firmly conclude that there are sleep traits. Do they make a difference? Certainly one of the differences that arises from variations among individuals relating to sleep length is a mischievous one resulting from a failure to recognize these natural divergencies. This emerges from a belief or a desire that everyone sleep the same amount. This in turn seems to be related to the unhealthy but natural human tendency to confuse an average with "normality." In study after study the *average* amount of sleep of adult humans, across a wide range of conditions and cultures, is seven to eight hours. This average becomes converted into a mythical norm.

It is not unusual for a sleep expert to be questioned as follows: "I sleep only six hours per night (or nine hours per night). Is this all right?" This problem is compounded by parents in relation to children, as we have seen in the chapter on age. Having in mind some implicit or explicit ideas about their child's need for sleep, parents faced with an unusually long or short sleep pattern do battle with nature. Even in adults, real problems can result from these differences. A marriage between a natural long sleeper and a natural short sleeper can run into problems. When one spouse needs to go to bed at 10 and the other at 2, and this happens nightly, problems can arise.

But what of more fundamental differences? Are long sleepers and short sleepers different from others in dimensions other than their sleep tendencies? There is disagreement on this question. Dr. Ernest Hartmann, a psychiatrist, holds that natural short sleepers are psychologically healthier than long sleepers. Short sleepers show traits of efficiency, ambitiousness, self-confidence, and high energy; and long sleepers have traits of depression, anxiety, and neuroticism. These conclusions were primarily adduced from interviews, since his objective test data on long sleepers and short sleepers revealed minimal differences. On the other hand, two studies in our laboratories failed to turn up any differences between "normal, young, healthy adults" who were long sleepers or short sleepers on objective measures of intelligence, personality, or general health. One thing is certain within this controversy. If differences are associated with different sleep lengths, they are by no means clear-cut or obvious.

We would hasten to emphasize that these findings refer to stable and natural individual differences. As we shall see in Chapter 12, a long or normal-length sleeper cannot simply become a short sleeper without consequences. Extreme state conditions (pathologies), such as psychoses or diseases, can increase or decrease sleep length. Such factors will be discussed later in this chapter.

The relationship between other traits and the substructural aspects of sleep is even less certain. So far as I know, no study has reported systematic relationships with the two variables that give evidence of being sleep-trait variables—Stage 4 and Stage 1. It is "rumored" that athletes tend to have high Stage 4 amounts. By "rumored" I mean that experienced sleep researchers have asystematically noticed this in their recording while doing other experiments. There has been a report of a relationship with a subcharacteristic of REM—the density of number of eye movements per unit time. These are significantly more in nonrecallers of dreams.

Where do these differences arise from? In regard to sleep length a highly probable source is stable differences between individuals in their inheritances. Genetics or heredity is the prime source of individual differences in traits that are heavily physiologically determined—height, weight, foot size, intelligence, and motor skills. Since sleep is certainly a biological system, it would follow that genetics is involved. This assumption is well supported by animal studies that show systematic sleep-length differences as a result of selective breeding.

These biological substrata involving the central nervous system and biochemical substrata that may be related to differences in sleep length can be "made" different by other variables than heredity. For example, we are increasingly aware of the often permanent effects of drugs. Other effects include poor nutrition and/or illness in the prenatal period, and good or bad nutrition, illness, or lack of illness and environmental impoverishment or enrichment during early development. It is reasonable to suppose that these factors, affecting the biophysiological substrata of the developing person, may result in differences in sleep.

Some differences in sleep length may be psychologically determined. This is apparent in all of us over short periods of time; voluntarily or under impositions of demands and stress (or lack thereof) we may, for varying periods of time, become short or long sleepers. It is possible that our early environmental conditioning by parental or cultural or circumstantial determinants may shape our later sleep patterns. It is not hard to believe that two children brought up to believe and forced to conform to a pattern of sleep that implied in one case that sleep was "vital" and in the other that it was "wasteful" would exhibit opposite sleep patterns.

Traits as determinants of sleep

Are there certain traits or differences among individuals that make for differences in sleep? We have, of course, touched on this question already by looking at differences in sleep as they are associated with different traits. But let us reexamine the issue by turning the question a full 180 degrees. Do different types of people sleep differently?

We are faced with a situation similar to that seen in our preceding chapter on precursors: the data is limited; the general effects seem slight within "normal" ranges; however, effects are likely between extreme differences.

Again the limited data is understandable. Such studies require a selection of presumed effective variables from an almost infinite variety of choices—height, weight, intelligence, creativity, aggressiveness, introversion, ad infinitum. These traits, particularly within the personality sphere, require accurate and effective definition and measurement. A large population should be measured. The sleep variables must be selected and then measured for this differentiated population. Sleep length must be defined by questionnaires or less dubious diaries, or all-night EEG recording must be undertaken for a number of nights.

However, as noted in relation to the precursors of sleep, we do have considerable data on a highly relevant set of individual differences: sex classification. At least at the time of the studies, men and women certainly had different traits. Study after study of both sleep-length variables and substructure characteristics have failed to find any remarkable or consistent differences between the sleep of males and females up to the age of about 50. If we are willing to accept certain population physiological differences, and perhaps some temperament differences, then these differences can be considered essentially independent of sleep behavior.

One study of more specific attributes or traits seems generally supportive of this independence of general traits and sleep traits. In a study of over 500 persons who kept sleep diaries for eight weeks it was found that neither a neuroticism scale nor an introversion scale was related to sleep length below the age of 40. (Beyond 40, introverts tended to have shorter sleep, which was contrary to the earlier findings reported above by Hartmann.) Similarly, in a study of over 100 medical students no scales on the MMPI—a personality test having some 13 subscales—were related to self-reported sleep length. As previously noted regarding long sleepers and short sleepers, we found no differences in their personality characteristics on an extensive battery of personality tests, and those reported by Hartmann were quite marginal and dubious. The previously mentioned study of the student group at the University of Florida also measured personality traits but produced no substantial relations with any sleep stage differences (Chapter 5).

What about intelligence? Does sleep length vary with being bright or dull (or vice versa)? The data suggests little or no relationship between intelligence and sleep length. A study of 509 "men of distinction" gave an average sleep period of 7.4 hours. We found no differences in aptitude tests or high school grades between long and short sleepers. Of considerable significance is the fact that essentially no difference in sleep stages has been found in mental retardates without central nervous system anomalies and individuals with normal or very high intelligence.

In short, the available evidence indicates that sleep pays little attention to whether we are males or females, tall or short, bright or dull, likable, hostile, shy, etc. It does not seem likely that less marked traits such as variations in introversion-extroversion, aggressiveness-passivity, being so smart or not being smart will make much greater difference in sleep.

We must add, as in our previous chapter, that extremes of traits are certainly likely to be interactive with sleep. There can be little doubt that being 9 feet tall or 400 pounds fat will certainly at least affect the logistics of sleeping. More seriously, however, we shall see in subsequent chapters that pathological conditions such as permanent brain damage, physiological debility, or psychopathology will affect sleep in specific ways. Similarly, it is likely that extreme maintained sleep traits are likely to affect behavior and result in stable differences. A person who sleeps chronically only 3 or 4 hours per day must be behaving consistently differently from a person sleeping 10 to 12 hours per day. Seven to nine hours of difference in amount of living should cause some stable differences in life-styles to accrue. Furthermore, we know that individuals sleep poorly or well across a broad range of adequacy. We will discuss these differences in the chapter on insomnia. Again, we must believe that chronic patterns of poor or good sleep at the extreme will result in consistent differences among people.

Implications

It is clear that there are stable differences among individuals in relation to the sleep characteristic. People sleep different lengths of time and people sleep differently within those lengths of time. However, it appears within a broad range which can be considered "normal" that these differences do not seem directly related to major differences in physiology, personality, or performance. It seems that just as there are people with large and small ears, there are natural long and short sleepers, and such differences may have as little influence on (or be the result of) other traits as differences in ear size or hair color.

8

The disorders of sleep

To this point we have reviewed the nature of natural or "normal" sleep and the variations imposed on it by everyday life: age, time variations, day-to-day variations in our activities, the environment, and inherent individual differences. In the next four chapters we will turn to the more unusual and extreme variations of sleep. In this chapter we will consider the distortions of sleep itself—disturbances of the primary sleep process. This will be followed by a chapter on the variations of sleep associated with pathologies of the brain, physiological disturbances, and psychopathology. We then turn to the great modern "distorter," the effects of drugs on sleep. Somewhat as a summarizing chapter in this series, we shall face the many faces of insomnia.

Specifically, in this chapter we are concerned with the primary sleep disorders and the parasomnias. These are disorders in which unusual sleep behaviors are the predominant symptoms of the disturbance. Two of the primary sleep disorders, narcolepsy, or "sleep attacks," and hypersomnia, or "excessive sleep," are sleep-"intrusive" disturbances in which the presence of sleep invades the waking state. Night terrors and nightmares, also classified as primary sleep disorders, are awake-"intrusive" disturbances in which waking behavior disturbs the sleep. The parasomnias refer to normal waking behavior appearing within the sleep and include sleepwalking, sleeptalking, and enuresis, or bed-wetting.

The primary sleep disorders

Narcolepsy (*narco* = "numbness"; *lepsy* = "seizure") is the most dramatic intrusion of sleep into the waking life. It is the presence of brief recurring, uncontrollable episodes of sleep during waking time. These are sometimes called "sleep attacks." The term was first used and clinical designation given to the condition in the 1880s and it has received intensive study in recent years. People with narcolepsy will, while performing normal day-to-day activities, suddenly and involuntarily lapse into sleep lasting from a very few minutes to episodes of up to 15 minutes. In addition to the overwhelming presence of sleep there are three additional symptoms that often accompany the attacks and have been called the "narcolepsy triad." In about 70 percent of the episodes there is a *catalepsy,* or muscular weakness, which may range from subjective feelings of weakness to total inability to move. A frequent accompaniment is *sleep paralysis,* which is a complete loss of muscle tone in the transition between sleep and waking and, less often, on awakening. This may be merely a focal aspect of catalepsy. Finally, somewhat more than 50 percent of the episodes will be associated with *hypnogogic hallucinations,* that is, unusual visual or auditory sensations at the onset of the attack.

It is estimated that between two to five persons in a thousand have narcoleptic episodes. The clinical case will typically have one to several episodes of daytime sleepiness per day, although in some cases the attacks will be less frequent. Generally, the person can "ward off" the attacks in dangerous situations, but occasionally this is not possible. Attacks are often precipitated by a heightened emotional response such as laughter or anger, but their likelihood also increases in conditions of fatigue or after heavy meals. About 75 percent of the attacks begin between the ages of 15 to 25. Some 5 percent may begin before the age of 10, but onset is rare after the age of 40.

The cause or causes of narcolepsy have not yet been clearly established. The recent work has, in general, disassociated narcolepsy from its earlier presumed relationship to epilepsy. There is no similarity of the EEG during the two attacks; narcolepsy shows typical sleep EEG tracings while epilepsy shows radically altered discharges. There is strong evidence of a hereditary or genetic component. Between 20 to 50 percent of diagnosed cases show the presence of narcolepsy in other family members. In general, the case for narcolepsy being of psychic origin is not strong. Two intensive and independent studies—one of 155 and the other of over 200 cases—lead both investigators to conclude that there was no evidence that their samples showed any specifically identifiable psychological dysfunctioning.

EEG research on narcoleptics has, however, established a clear-cut relationship between narcoleptic attacks and REM sleep. It will be recalled that in normal sleep, REM episodes rarely occur before about 60 to 90 minutes of sleep. Further note that REM episodes, particularly in lower animals, are associated with a cataplexy, or sleep paralysis, and, in human subjects, with "dreamlike" mental content. In a systematic study of 49 narcoleptics showing one or more of the narcoleptic triad (cataplexy, paralysis, and hypnogogic hallucinations), 90 percent of the patients showed REM sleep episodes at the onset of their daytime sleep periods. In short, there is strong evidence, confirmed by a number of other studies, that narcolepsy may well be considered a REM dysfunction disorder and that this may account for its symptoms.

We are at the point where narcolepsy can be specifically diagnosed. In many instances treatment with drugs directed at REM suppression has been found effective. Just as important, it is helpful for the person to understand his condition and his symptoms and to know that he is not psychotic, epileptic, or a freak. Rather, he simply suffers from attacks of sleep. Knowing this, inconvenient and even embarrassing as the attacks may be, the person can adjust to them in a healthy and essentially normal way.

Hypersomnia (*hyper* = "excessive"; *somnia* = "sleep") refers to sleep in excessive amounts within each 24 hours. This may take the form of extended sleep periods or extreme drowsiness during the normal waking period. It should be emphasized that we are talking about sleep amounts beyond 12 hours per 24, which appear to be beyond the normal range of natural long sleepers.

The most prevalent hypersomnias are those associated with pathological brain conditions and are discussed in the next chapter on secondary sleep disorders. The "functional," or "idiopathic," hypersomnias are rare. In the reported cases that have been studied, however, hypersomniacs show distinct differences from narcoleptics. They show a large amount of slow-wave (Stages 3–4) sleep and a relatively low amount of REM sleep. While narcoleptics frequently have complaints about nighttime sleep, the hypersomniacs may complain about sleeping "too deeply." They are difficult to awaken and may show confusion, disorientation, and sleepiness for an hour or more after awakening. Their daytime naps will be longer than the more typical 30 to 60 minutes, and such naps will not be refreshing.

Little is known about the etiology of hypersomnia and it is

important in diagnosis to rule out organic disorders or narcolepsy. The use of stimulants is often helpful in symptom relief.

Night terrors and nightmares are episodes of awakening from sleep in a state of anxiety. They are distinct from each other and also from the common experience of simply waking up and recalling an unpleasant dream. While the distinction between the nightmare and the bad dream may be merely one of degree, the former is characterized by abruptness and involuntary awakening.

Night terrors, technically known as *pavor nocturnus* (night fear), are most frequent between the ages of three to five. It is estimated that between 2 to 5 percent of all children may have one or more episodes during this period. They are characterized by an abrupt awakening from sleep, accompanied by extreme panic reactions. The child may scream and sit upright while staring wide-eyed and breathing rapidly. There is every physical evidence of extreme fright.

Night terrors differ from nightmares in several distinct ways. The child reports no frightening thoughts or dreams in association with these awakenings. After returning to sleep the child typically does not remember the episode in the morning. This lack of frightening mental content is reasonable since night terrors do not emerge from REM or dream sleep but are arousals from slow-wave (Stage 4) sleep, during which little or no mental content is present. Simply, night terrors do not result from bad dreams but are awakenings from very deep sleep. The terror probably stems from the rapid and radical shift in the level of consciousness—being tossed suddenly from a "nonworld" into a "waking world."

Although these episodes may be repeated in some children, they have seldom been reported as chronic or persistent occurrences and typically disappear without treatment. They have not been associated with particular presleep circumstances or personality traits. In short, while they are likely to be terrifying to concerned parents, they appear to be a momentary and apparently unconscious part of the child's concern. The best treatment seems to be a calm reassurance of the child at the time.

Nightmares peak somewhat later, between the ages of seven and ten. These are awakenings accompanied by frightening dream recalls and do evolve from "bad dreams" associated with REM sleep. The child, on awakening, reports having been frightened by something in his dreams. While the awakening somatic anxiety responses are far less than those associated with the night terrors, the consciousness of being frightened is often elaborated and extended into the now waking world and the entire environment is reacted to with fright. In these cases, the child needs considerable reassurance, particularly if he is a very young child, and a distinction between the dream world and the real world needs emphasis.

Some 5 percent of parents report the presence in their children of intermittent nightmares so extensive as to cause them concern. It is likely that a preponderance of these episodes does represent a reaction to some "pressure" in the child's life. The wise parent should view these as such signals. However, the sources are not likely to be simple or readily interpreted. A child's view of the world and his definition of pressures are likely to be quite different from ours. Again, these episodes appear to be intermittent rather than chronic and have not been associated with any psychopathological condition with any certainty. They do not appear to be true dysfunctions of sleep but extensions of the normal. Unless they are chronic and disturbing to the child's general adjustment they are best viewed as a part of growing up.

In some few instances, night terrors and nightmares persist into adulthood. In these cases they do probably represent dysfunctions of the sleep process; slow-wave dysfunctions in the case of night terrors and REM sleep dysfunctions in the case of nightmares. Some success has been had in treatment with the use of drugs that specifically depress slow-wave or REM sleep.

Finally, one specific cause of nightmares deserves special mention. We shall see that nightmares are a predictable and common concomitant of withdrawal from drugs. This will be discussed in the chapter on drugs and sleep.

The parasomnias

The parasomnias (*para* = "akin to"; *somnia* = "sleep") include a group of "wakelike" behaviors that intrude into or occur during sleep. The most prominent of these are somnambulism (*somnus* = "sleep"; *ambulus* = "walk") or sleepwalking, sleeptalking, and enuresis (Greek: *enourein* = "urinate in bed") or bed-wetting.

In the literature, as late as the 1960s the striking phenomenon of sleepwalking was variously interpreted as a neurotic symptom, a hysterical reaction, a disassociated personality state and, in particular, an acting out of dreams. These viewpoints stemmed primarily from clinical practice and secondhand reports. Laboratory studies of the phenomenon have resulted in the more benign viewpoint that sleepwalking is a sleep disorder that may or may not be associated with other pathological conditions. It has been clearly demonstrated that sleepwalking is not a walking dream state. Rather, sleepwalking is associated with slow-wave sleep (Stage 4) and not the REM state of sleep associated with dreaming.

During a sleepwalking episode movements tend to be restricted to more "automatic" behaviors and the person has a low reactivity to the environment around him. Awakening is typically difficult and the person is usually in a confused state. He has no dream recall. If not fully awakened the person is amnesic for the entire event. The episodes may be quite brief and limited to getting up, standing briefly, and then returning to bed. They may be more extended: getting up and going to the door, or getting partially dressed, or going to sleep on a couch. Less frequently (though more frequently reported or commented on) the episodes may be more extended or complex: going to the kitchen and getting out pans, getting into a car, or walking in the yard. Because movements may be repetitive and "inner-controlled," they may be viewed as ritualistic. Dr. Seuss has illustrated the sleepwalking of the Hoop-Soup-Snoop Group.

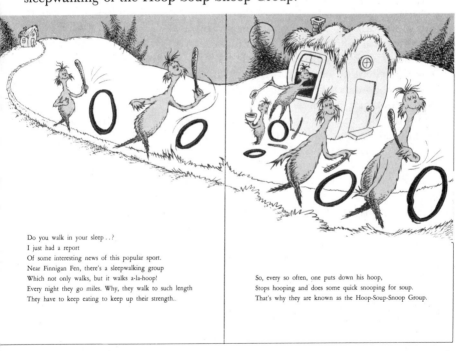

Do you walk in your sleep ..?
I just had a report
Of some interesting news of this popular sport.
Near Finnigan Fen, there's a sleepwalking group
Which not only walks, but it walks a-la-hoop!
Every night they go miles. Why, they walk to such length
They have to keep eating to keep up their strength..

So, every so often, one puts down his hoop,
Stops hooping and does some quick snooping for soup.
That's why they are known as the Hoop-Soup-Snoop Group.

Sleepwalking may vary from once in a lifetime to every night and may disappear with age. As noted above, the range of behavior is from limited movements to very elaborate excursions. As such the amount of sleepwalking is difficult to assess. One or two episodes may worry certain parents and many episodes may never be observed. However, it appears that between 10–20 percent of people questioned can recall one or more sleepwalking episodes. Some 5 percent of a college population described themselves as "sleepwalkers" without defining recency or severity. Sleepwalking tends to peak in early adolescence (9–12 years old) and diminish thereafter. It may occur in adulthood, but typically as only a rare episode. It is clearly episodic—that is, it seldom is seen as a persistent nightly condition.

The cause of sleepwalking is by no means certain. Explanations relative to neuroticism or organic conditions such as epilepsy or immaturity have been made uncertain by studies that have failed to find a consistent relationship to such conditions. One thing may be said with certainty. This is not an acting out of dreams or the result of some specific psychic dream pressure. All laboratory studies have consistently confirmed the fact that sleepwalking occurs in Stage 4 or deep sleep, not in REM or dream sleep. One association seems persistent: genetic and familial disposition. Several studies have found that sleepwalking seems to run in families. There is good evidence to indicate that sleepwalking is associated with other sleep anomalies, particularly those of the "deep sleep" kind such as night terrors and, to a lesser extent, enuresis and sleeptalking.

In a sleepwalking episode the possibility of harm to the individual should not be minimized. Simply, when such episodes are persistent, doors should be locked. Within an episode an individual can usually be guided to bed and can certainly be awakened. If, however, the person is awakened he is likely to be confused and will need reassurance.

Sleeptalking, while a disturbance threatening only the sleeping companion, has intrigued sleep researchers as an avenue to the sleeper's consciousness. Unfortunately, little of value has resulted from this interest. Most sleeptalking does not occur in REM sleep. Because there are many EEG artifacts associated with sleeptalking it is difficult to assess the precise non-REM stage, but the best evidence is that it occurs in Stage 1 or even Stage 0. In short, the individual is in a borderline state between sleep and waking. This makes it easy to understand why the sleeptalker can often be "talked with." Because he is partially awake, this contact is possible; because he is partially asleep, the response is often "suggestible" and "free." However, sleeptalking does occur occasionally in Stage REM or dream sleep. In one laboratory study this occurred in 10 percent of the episodes observed. The character of talking from REM sleep typically shows an emotional quality and there is usually no reference point in the surround. If the person awakens or is awakened, the talking is often clearly related to dream content. This is in contrast to the non-REM talk which is less emotional, situationally related, and on awakening presents no recall of dreams.

Bed-wetting or enuresis as a sleep problem is by far the most common of the sleep anomalies that we have discussed. As with the other disorders, persistence and frequency are problems in defining the extent of the disorder as well as the level of reaction by either the individual or his parents. In this particular problem there is the further difficulty of setting the age after which bed-wetting should be considered a "disorder" in contrast to simply a delayed maturation. Three years old is typically cited as the average age of bladder control throughout the night. However, because this is an average, bed-wetting up to at least the age of four is seldom considered a clinical case of enuresis. In a large sample of children between the ages of 4 and 14 there was a reported 29 percent incidence in recent bed-wetting. The majority of the cases were in the 5, 6 and 7 year old groups. The number reduced sharply with age. There was, however, a persistence in the older sample with about 1 percent reporting some bed-wetting in the 14-year-old group. The incidence was significantly greater among boys than girls.

EEG studies have been less clear in their association of sleep stages with bed-wetting but the preponderance of the data associates the event with non-REM sleep. Some authors equate it with slow-wave disturbances. It is clear that bed-wetting seldom occurs during REM sleep episodes although it may precede and follow such episodes. The individual may have wet the bed prior to the REM episode and on awakening from the REM state may have incorporated the wetness of the bed into his dream content.

In terms of etiology, early notions concentrating almost exclusively on pathological or psychopathological or neurotic causes have markedly abated. Studies implicating genetics, maturational rates, psychogenesis, or poor habit-training as well as specific neurological and urological disorders have been found to be factors in some cases but not in others. It is most likely that one or more of these factors may be the specific cause of any particular case. Further, there have been a variety of attempts at control, including conditioning, liquid intake control, psychotherapy, and drugs. These have met with varying reports of success, with the likelihood of success being dependent upon the matching of cause and the cure.

Because of the complexity of etiology, and particularly because of shame, guilt, and anxiety on the part of both parents and the child, first efforts should be directed to not overreacting to the inconvenience involved. In the face of real persistence, and an expressed concern of the child (typically in the form of social inconvenience), expert help should be sought.

Implications

Difficulties associated with any pathological conditions, whether they be physiological or psychological, are that they lend themselves to self-diagnosis or, in the case of children, to parental diagnosis. This often results in a normal, simple, variation being exaggerated into a presumed pathology with all of the accompanying anxiety. On the other hand, the real presence of an anomaly, if ignored or lived with under considerable stress, may result in an untreated but treatable condition, or a misunderstanding or exaggeration of a condition that deserves far less concern than it causes.

9

Sleep and pathological conditions

The sleep that we have discussed so far has, on the whole, been a sturdy process that naturally unfolds according to its own nature. While showing some responsiveness to conditions of age, timing, precursors, and environment, the structure has been one that primarily struggles to maintain its integrity. The anomalies are relatively rare and often outgrown. In this chapter we will briefly review the system of sleep under the extreme pressures of pathological conditions. These disturbances of sleep have been classified as the *secondary sleep disorders,* in which sleep variations are secondary accompaniments of primary pathological states. We have divided these conditions into neuropathological, physiopathological, and psychopathological.

These are clinical disorders that require specific and specialized treatment. We can do little ourselves to control them. Nevertheless, they deserve our attention. At a practical level, disturbed sleep is a prominent accompaniment of a number of pathological conditions. A sensitivity to this may help us to better understand the behavior of individuals suffering from these disorders. We may recognize that, in their presence, the sufferer is more than simply upset or anxious—he cannot, in fact, perform the act of sleeping. Further, if we can observe sleep-related responses to these particular and extreme conditions, we may better understand the mechanisms of sleep itself. In this sense, pathological conditions can be viewed as "experiments in nature." For example, if we wish to know the relationship between waking hallucinations and dreams, what better way than by observing this relationship in active hallucinators?

Neurological pathologies

The brain, or central nervous system, is where the primary mechanisms of sleep are deeply embedded. There have been and continue to be a large number of clinical reports of the relationship between brain dysfunctions and sleep, since variations in sleep are quite prominent in central nervous system pathologies. The earlier approach to an understanding of sleep and the brain was almost exclusively dependent upon these clinical observations. This approach today has been largely superseded by studies with animals, in which lesions and electrical and chemical stimulations are specifically controlled and electrophysiological measures are made down to the single nerve cell.

Figure 9-1 presents a very simplified schematic of the brain. This area can become "pathological" in five general ways: by infection; by tumors or growths; by trauma or physical impact; by vascular changes; by deterioration. Each of these neurological variations have particularized characteristics in terms of extensity, probable site, rate of onset, and rate of progress. The resultant associated sleep disturb-

Fig. 9-1   A schematic diagram of the human brain.

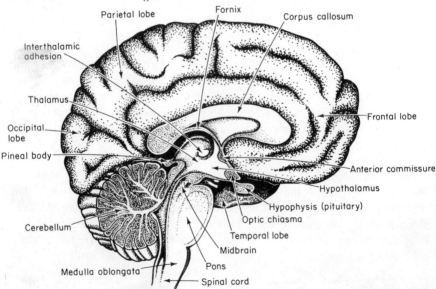

ances are dependent on all of these variations, with particular emphasis on the locus and extensity of the change.

One infectious invasion of the central nervous system results in such dramatic changes in sleeping that it is commonly known as "sleeping sickness," or *encephalitis lethargica.* This is apparently a viral infection with a particular affinity for the hypothalamic region (see figure 9-1). There have been a number of epidemic outbursts of encephalitis lethargica; there was a particularly severe one in Italy in the winter of 1919–20 and in St. Louis in the mid 1920s. This disorder is carried by the tsetse fly in Africa and is quite prevalent on that continent. There is first a high fever, followed by a hyperactive state lasting for as long as six weeks and finally a cessation of the fever with a residual hypersomnia, or excessive sleep. This excessive sleep appears essentially normal. It differs from a stupor because the person can be aroused from the sleep to alertness but cannot maintain wakefulness.

The effects of tumors and other neoplasms, or growths, on sleep are various and complex due to wide differences in their placement and size. The matter is further complicated by the fact that increased intracranial pressure is present in most cases and hence the growth may extend its influence, by pressure, beyond its site onto other structures. Moreover, it is often difficult to distinguish between a stupor or coma and an increased tendency to sleep. Nevertheless, some generalizations can be made. Hyposomnia, or reduced sleep, is seldom seen in such cases. Surprisingly large growths may have no effect on sleep and waking patterns if there is limited intracranial pressure. This is particularly true of frontal or temporal involvements. In one study of temporal-lobe tumors only 9 of 38 cases showed hypersomnia. However, growths in the thalamic and hypothalamic regions frequently show a hypersomnia. In a summary of cases involving these areas, some 40 percent of the cases had symptoms of hypersomnia or stupor.

Head traumas may, of course, be of varying severity and may injure various parts of the brain. This is usually by a direct "compacting" of the brain against its encasing, but there may be a direct lesion of the brain by breaking through the skull or an involvement of the blood supply of the brain. A severe head blow may result in a deep coma. Recent studies of the EEG of traumatized patients in comas have yielded interesting results. In many patients, the sleep/waking rhythm is maintained. While some patients may show this by the presence of sleep spindles or even a simple "fast-slow" wave change or differential flattening of the nocturnal EEG, some other patients in deep stuporous or semicomatose states may display a relatively intact sleep pattern. Most recent evidence has suggested this latter to be a favorable prognostic sign.

There is no reported data on the effects of sleep of sudden vascular changes in the brain resulting, for example, from an aneurysm, or "stroke." The effects are likely to be quite varied and dependent upon extensity and site of the aneurysm, the absorption and the development or presence of collateral blood supply.

There are deteriorative or degenerative changes in the central nervous system associated with aging. These changes are, of course, a matter of degree over time and different among individuals. Further, it is quite likely that there may be a specificity of rate of deterioration in different brain areas. Where the changes are extensive they result in behavioral disturbances, and extreme changes are classified as "psychoses" (see next section).

We have reviewed the general effects of aging on sleep in a previous chapter: sleep becomes more fragmented, Stage 4 sleep is sharply diminished, with only limited losses of REM sleep. However, more extreme brain deterioration typically has sharp and distinct effects on sleep. A group of patients classified Chronic Brain Syndrome cases were studied. These are patients in which the aging process (particularly associated with cognitive functioning) has been accentuated and has resulted in a severely demented condition. They were compared with an age-matched group of healthy elderly subjects. They had less sleep, longer latencies to sleep, and more wakefulness during sleep. These may be simply an extension of the aging process. They showed a sharp decrease in REM sleep amounts generally exceeding that expected from the reduced sleep length.

Illnesses and general physiological pathologies

Illnesses and general physiological dysfunctions such as digestive, vascular, or glandular difficulties may affect sleep. Sleep also may have an effect in relation to these disorders. There have, however, been few studies of these effects. This is probably due to several reasons. In acute illnesses, the focus is on the treatment of the particular problem. In the face of pneumonia or an appendicitis, sleep is of secondary concern. Sleep often has no relevance to the illness or disorder except as indirectly associated with the anxiety involved. If there is a heart condition, or glaucoma, or diabetes, for example, "How are you sleeping?" does not follow logically as a question. In many illnesses the patient is confined to his bed and sleep may be presumed to be sufficient. In a number of illnesses and disorders, however, sleep disturbances are common clinical manifestations. In others, such as thyroid disorders, the relationship to sleep is logical. In still others, sleep may be suspect in its role in exaggerating the disorder.

An elevated body temperature is a frequent accompaniment of illness and has an effect on sleep. In less than extreme ranges (studies have not been conducted at the very high level of temperature) sleep becomes fragmented, with increased number of awakenings and some reduction in both slow-wave sleep and REM sleep. It is not known whether the total amount of sleep within 24 hours is reduced or increased, but it is likely that at least the reduced sleep obtained during the night is distributed into the day period resulting in "dozing" and napping. Because a lower temperature is a natural part of the biorhythm of sleep it is generally thought that the effect of the increased temperature on sleep during the sleep period is a result of the disruption of this biorhythm.

Poor sleep during the night, often accompanied by drowsiness during the day, is a frequently reported pattern in cases of renal, or kidney, disorders. This pattern may be similar in form and cause to that of the temperature findings since there is a biorhythm of urine output associated with the sleep/wake rhythm. EEG studies have confirmed the reduced total sleep, increased awakening, and lowered slow-wave sleep. The two studies of patients maintained on artificial kidneys are in conflict, since one showed no sleep disturbances while the other showed some continuing disturbances. A kidney transplant study showed a continued sleep disturbance and it was argued that this may be evidence for an irreversible damage to the sleep mechanism.

Because an over- or underproduction of thyroid affects general activity levels during the waking hours, several studies have evaluated sleep in such cases. Hyperthyroid (excess thyroid) cases did indeed show light, fragmented sleep with very little slow-wave sleep. Hypothyroid (insufficient thyroid) infants showed a reduced "spindle" activity, which was interpreted as a sign of retarded central nervous system development. Hypothyroid adult patients had essentially normal EEG patterns of sleep with some lowering of slow-wave sleep amounts. Under treatment these patients showed an increase in slow-wave sleep.

The effect of sleep on several physiological disturbances has been studied. A common complaint of duodenal ulcer patients is gastric pain and awakening from sleep. It has been found that gastric secretion is 3 to 20 times in excess of normal subjects and that marked increases are directly related to REM episodes in sleep. Cardiovascular disturbances are also exacerbated during REM sleep periods. This has been established in regard to angina pains, myocardial infarctions, and migraine headaches. A very recent set of studies of apnea, or breathing difficulties, has shown a clear-cut relationship between respiration and 'sleep. It would seem that the control of breathing is less effective during sleep than during waking.

The young science of sleep has just begun to explore the interrelations between physiological disorders and sleep. All of the studies reported have been conducted since the 1960's. As one clinician put it, ". . . if the treatment of many disorders is not based on sleeping as well as the waking behavior of the patient, then it is only partial treatment."

The psychopathologies

Definitions are always a problem and in this area they are rampant. When we refer to psychopathological conditions we generally refer to behavior that is extreme—overreactions, underreactions, or disorganized behavior for which no physiological basis can be found and for which a psychological cause is presumed. The psychological causes of these behaviors may be subdivided into those externally generated and those internally generated. External causes are responses generated by the environment that exceed the person's capacity to cope effectively. These demands stem from emergencies, continued pressures, or severe losses and the like—factors which we discussed in the earlier chapter on precursors of sleep. The internally generated psychopathologies are generally subdivided into the neuroses and the psychoses.

THE NEUROSES AND SLEEP

The neuroses, often resulting from an interplay between personal inadequacies and persistent environmental pressures, are troublesome enough to limit the person's effective functioning in his day-to-day affairs and require expert help. They only occasionally require hospitalization. They are attempts to cope with persistent conflicts. Anxiety is the most prominent symptom of the neuroses, but their expression may involve obsessive-compulsive behavior (repetitious and rigid thoughts and acts), phobic responses (focused extreme fears), or conversion reactions. These latter are "conversions" of the problem to physical symptoms for which there are no underlying physical causes: vague aches and pains, listlessness, or even paralysis.

In a review article on neuroses it was reported that 50 percent of neurotics complained of insomnia. It is surprising that the figure is not higher. In the earlier chapter on precursors of sleep we concluded that circumstances which promoted a persistent demand for continued response would disrupt sleep and that the stronger these tendencies were, the greater the likelihood of sleep disturbance. Neurotics are persons deeply troubled by their inability to cope with persistent conflicts; under continuous pressure, their defense against these pressures could hardly promote sleep.

A considerable number of case reports and clinical observations provide an elaboration of this reasoning. Sleep is again and again seen as disrupted by real, imagined, or exaggerated responses to threatening aspects of the environment. Sleep is held off by these defenses and, once asleep, the person continues to be threatened with consequent awakenings.

Psychoanalysts have emphasized the problems associated with the reduced levels of impulse control or defense at the outset of and during sleep itself. There is a resultant tendency for a "breakthrough" of prohibited impulses and feelings of guilt, hostility, and anxiety, and a subsequent interference with sleep. In one report an elderly unmarried woman is quoted: "I was very sleepy but I was afraid to fall asleep because when I dozed off I saw a pair of arms embracing me. I cried, 'No, no!'" Other analysts have posited or described problems associated with "separation anxieties," in which the person fears a loss or separation from the world he knows or from some supportive person. Still others have noted the interfering presence of defensive "obsessional" thinking: repeated nonthreatening thoughts to "hold off" disturbing or threatening thoughts and impulses.

There is certainly the possibility of "vicious circling," particularly in neurotics with hypochondriacal or "conversion" tendencies. Sleeping poorly may result in feeling poorly during the day. These general feelings of inadequate functioning and general malaise may become focal points of worry and a part of the defense system: "If only I could sleep I would be able to cope." Indeed, they may become a core of the neurotic defense and even become a needed part of that defense to the point of unconscious exaggeration. These worries then would be added to the interference pattern.

But could sleep itself not serve as a defense? Given an unpleasant world, could we not escape into sleep? Although there have been a few reports of "defensive" sleeping, it is not a common response to threat. There are some reports of sleeping during analytical sessions or even in the therapist's waiting room. In a few isolated cases increased sleep tendencies have been reported in response to severe and sustained threats or losses. Many of these instances may, however, be the result of prolonged lack of sleep or poor sleep prior to the event.

We will later argue that sleep did in fact evolve as a defense against a hostile environment. In its evolved form, however, it does not seem likely that the sleep will often occur readily or be a strong response tendency in the face of threatening circumstances of feelings of threat or danger. Rather, these are most likely to evoke defensive responses which are themselves incompatible with sleep. It is neither adaptive nor rational to lie down and sleep before real or imagined dangers. While one may run or hide from real threats or uncomfortable situations there is no hiding place from one's thoughts, and so long as they persist, sleep is unlikely.

Two reports from sleep clinics attest to the relationship between sleep disturbances and neuroticism. Both studies, one involving 30 and the other involving 124 chronic insomniacs, used the Minnesota Multiphasic test, which has a "neurotic triad." These are tendencies toward depression, hysteria, and hypochondrias (somatic conversions). In both samples these profiles were significantly elevated and were the single most predominant characteristic of the chronic insomniacs. A score of 70 on this test is considered in the pathological range. In the smaller sample 50 percent of the subjects exceeded 70 on these three scales; in the larger sample 61, 46, and 31 percent of the cases fell in the pathological range on depression, hysteria, and hypochondriasis respectively.

The psychoses and sleep

The psychoses are more severe behavior disorders that typically require hospitalization and may be psychogenic or organic in origin. The behavior is disorganized and social functioning is badly disrupted. The two most prominent psychoses, generally classified as psychogenic in origin, are the schizophrenias and manic-depressive reactions. The most numerous of the psychoses are associated with aging.

The symptoms of schizophrenia are widely varied but the primary syndrome includes some or all of the following symptoms: 1) A disturbed affect in the form of flattened or inappropriate emotional responses, 2) A loss of contact with "reality" or the world around one and a self-absorption in one's inner world, 3) Delusions or hallucinations, 4) Incoherent thought patterns and bizarre behavioral gestures or movements. The manic-depressive psychoses are characterized by recurrent and exaggerated swings of moods and associated behavior. This may take the form of either a manic, or overexcited response, or a depressive reaction with associated feeling of depression and reduced responsiveness. These states may alternate, take one form or the other, or combine in an "agitated" depression. The depressive reaction is the most common manifestation.

Distinctions between "normality" and psychopathology are not absolute or clear-cut, and the distinctions drawn within the psychopathologies both as to cause and degree are very arbitrary.

The relationships between sleep and schizophrenia and manic depression have been extensively explored. The impetus for these research efforts emerged from two different interests. The symptoms of schizophrenia, particularly the flattened or disassociated affect, the strange and bizarre gestures, and the hallucinatory behavior, had often been connected by analogy to dreaming. Among the earliest sleep studies after the discovery of REM sleep were those exploring this linkage. Interests in a possible connection between the manic-depressive psychoses and sleep reflected both a logical concern and clinical observations. Logically the question was whether the waking behavior carried over into sleep. Did the highly active and excited behavior of the manic result in less sleep? Did the slowed and depressed behavior of the depressive result in more sleep? Clinically the question was whether the common observation of poor sleep in most cases of depression is an essential part of the disorder and if so, to what extent.

The sleep of schizophrenic patients revealed startling findings. Their sleep was remarkably undisturbed. While disturbances could be found in acute and onset phase of schizophrenia, study after study found little difference in comparison of their sleep with that of normal control cases. Either an increase or a decrease in REM sleep would have been considered sensible. The former would have suggested a reduction in REM pressure in sleep due to the "dreamlike" hallucinatory and other schizophrenic waking behavior. The latter would have been explainable as a "spillover" REM "pressure." Recent evidence has indicated some depression of slow-wave sleep in schizophrenia but again the decrement is not excessive or beyond that seen in much less disturbed somato- or psychopathological conditions. This generally "normal" sleep in individuals who are clearly exhibiting highly distorted cognitive, emotional, and behavioral disturbances during their waking hours has done much to discourage hopes of finding significant presleep variables as strong determinates of the sleep structure (Chapter 6).

The sleep studies of manic-depressives have generally confirmed the clinical impressions of disturbed sleep. These patients during both manic and depressive episodes generally show long sleep latencies, shorter total sleep time, frequent awakening and, often, early awakenings. There is also typically a marked reduction in slow-wave sleep. Most studies have reported some reduction in REM time, although several have reported little or no change and two studies reported an actual increase. Several studies have established a clear-cut relationship between recovery from the psychoses and a parallel recovery of sleep patterns.

The largest number of psychoses are those associated with central nervous system degeneration due to aging. We have noted under the section on neuropathologies that those sleep disturbances naturally associated with aging are typical and exaggerated in these disorders, with some evidence of an excessive loss of REM sleep.

Implications

We have seen in this chapter the impact on sleep of extreme pressures. We reviewed the effects of neuropathological, physiopathological, and psychopathological conditions.

The "control" of sleep, in terms of underlying sleep mechanisms, is in the brain and damage to this system frequently results in disturbed sleep. However, because sleep mechanisms have specificity in the brain, the degree of disturbance is highly dependent upon both the extensiveness and the area of the involvement. Damage to or pressure upon the midbrain area, particularly involving the hypothalamus and the thalamic areas, shows the most marked effects, with a typical pattern of increased sleep. Surprisingly, extensive involvements outside these areas may have little effect on sleep. The extremes or acceleration of the deteriorative processes seen in normal aging show marked effects on sleep in the form of fragmented patterns of reduced sleep.

Clearly the influence on and influence of sleep extends beyond the central nervous system. Illnesses resulting in temperatures show disrupted sleep patterns. The effect on sleep may be an indirect one through the disruption of the biorhythmic substrata underlying sleep. Certain bodily dysfunctions in themselves have been found to disrupt sleep. Kidney disorders and thyroid malfunctioning are examples that have been studied. Most important, sleep has been found to exaggerate or dampen a broad range of physiological disorders such as ulcers and certain heart, respiratory, and vascular conditions. Truly to treat many pathophysiological conditions independent of sleep is to treat only partially those conditions.

The relationship between sleep and the psychopathologies is

particularly revealing. The manic-depressive psychoses sharply disrupt sleep. Inadequate or disturbed sleep is commonly associated with the psychoneuroses. The schizophrenics, presenting a picture of highly distorted thinking and emotional responses, show little or no change in sleep. Clearly, then, unusual thinking or emotional patterns in and of themselves are not essential determinants of sleep. The clue perhaps lies in the relationship of the behavior to the environment. The manic-depressive is overreacting to his environment. The psychoneurotic is defensively reacting to his persistent conflicts and problems. In contrast, the schizophrenic is essentially "disassociated," or withdrawn from the environment, and is reacting to a private world or "pseudocommunity." Within this world sleep drifts into its natural form.

10

Drugs and sleep

The relationship between drugs and any human functioning is almost inevitably balanced on a knife edge of promises and problems. Certainly this is the current status of drugs and sleep. On one side there is the promise of "sweet sleep" to be bought in troubled times and disordered states of mind. History, literature, folkways, and medical practice are rife with references to "sleeping potions" and the new world of pharmaceutical "magic" has accentuated this hope. To an increasingly complex battery of sedatives have now been added the "tranquilizers" and "antidepressants." In addition to this promise of inducing sleep, the promise of holding off sleep has received increased emphasis. The old standby of constant cups of coffee was joined by the World War II creation of powerful central nervous system stimulants such as amphetamine.

But with this promise there are associated problems. These extend far beyond the simple failure of the promise. In some instances the drugs used to aid sleep may actually distort the process of sleep severely. However, the major problems stem from the abuse of drugs and the resultant devastations to the sleep state.

A dramatic picture of the extensiveness of the problems associated with drugs and their intimate relationship to sleep was graphically written about by Luce and Segal in their book *Sleep* (New York: Coward-McCann). Since this book was published in 1966, we can only believe that the picture is even more accentuated today. Certainly there is no evidence to the contrary. As the authors state:

> Millions of Americans who would never dream of injecting themselves with heroin have recently begun to ply themselves with sedatives,

tranquilizers, alcohol and stimulants—casually and without apprehension. Many of these new drugs are invaluable in medicine. . . . In balance with their medical merit we now witness the gravity of careless handling and abuse, often arising from poor sleep habits or relatively mild sleep difficulties associated with psychological problems.

Doctors administer barbiturates to some twenty million patients each year, and stimulants such as dexedrine to about ten million . . . Americans pay about $100 million for prescription sedatives each year—about $350 million if over-the-counter drugs and hospital purchases are included. About $250 million are spent on tranquilizers, and the yearly purchase of America's foremost psychotoxic drug—alcohol—amounts to nearly $18 billion.

These figures barely suggest the extent to which drugs have been used to substitute for a well-balanced nervous system. The U.S. Food and Drug Administration has estimated that about half of our barbiturates and amphetamines are diverted from the legal market. We produce about 6 to 10 billion barbiturate capsules and 8 billion amphetamine capsules a year. Illegal traffic in "pep pills" alone amounts to something between $200 million and $400 million a year.

. . . the addict is quite likely to be a wealthy suburban housewife or a respected professional. For every person hooked on narcotics there are about twelve who are hooked on barbiturates. . . . Sleeping pills are abused and illegally purchased in every level of society. . . . Widely dispensed by doctors, accepted in society, these medical drugs are considered safe and comfortable—assurances of needed sleep, calmed nerves, a backstop of alertness and courage for long stretches of duty. . . .

Inordinate reliance on drugs is kindled by a slow and beguiling process. Amphetamines and barbiturates develop tolerances in the individual, which is to say that the body adjusts to repeated doses so that they no longer instigate their original effects. . . . When a person takes a sleeping pill . . . [the] tolerance mechanism slowly diminishes the effect so that he is forced to take ever more. Millions of people drift down this path so gently they do not realize what may be happening to them (pp. 141–144).

There are more than 60 prescription sedatives, most of which are "sleeping pills." In addition, there are more than 200 prescription tranquilizers and antidepressants, and a narrower range of stimulants which are often implicated in the "control" of sleep. There are a variety of "over-the-counter" (nonprescription) "sleeping aids" such as Sominex, Nytol, and Sleep-Eze. Finally, there is our major uncontrolled sedative and stimulant pair: alcohol and caffeine.

The study of drugs and sleep

There has been an increasing number of laboratory studies of the effects of the various drugs on sleep. These are very complicated experiments to conduct and involve requirements of many safeguards in their design and decisions about subjects and dosage. We will concentrate on those that have been conducted in laboratories and which utilized the EEG. In these, at least, the specific effects on the sleep process are carefully assessed.

The simplest requirement involves the use of a "double-blind" procedure. These experiments require the use of a "placebo," a pill identical to that being tested but containing an inert or nonactive substance. In the double-blind procedure neither the patient nor the experimenter knows the occasion on which the drug rather than the placebo is being administered. This procedure is an attempt to separate the element of "suggestion" about the efficacy of the drug from its physiological action. Of course, this procedure often is not completely foolproof since the drug may have a clearly discernible effect, in which case the patient knows that he has taken the drug and not the placebo and, as a consequence, the matter of "expectancies" is back in the picture.

A most difficult problem is the selection of the subject population. To evaluate realistically a drug's clinical effectiveness one might wish to select insomniacs to see if the drug will be helpful to those who need it most. However, as we shall see in the following chapter, a population of insomniacs is a heterogeneous mixture of symptoms and causes in varying degrees of chronicity and severity of symptoms. A drug that may be effective for one portion of this mixed population may be completely ineffective for another group. The insomnia may be simply a secondary symptom of a more primary cause totally irrelevant to the drug used. Moreover, the "hard-core" insomniac may well have a long and/or current drug history as a result of his past attempts to cope with his complaint.

On the other hand, the use of "normal" or untroubled sleepers has its limitations. The variables of latency and awakenings that are of particular interest are likely to be very low, with little improvement possible. Most critically, the clinician will be very cautious about putting individuals on a drug routine for an extended period of time lest the experiment itself encourage the development of a drug dependency. Thus, findings about tolerance and withdrawal effects will be quite limited.

The best studies are those which establish a "dosage effect," or differential response to the amount of the drug used. A typical base level of the drug would be the "clinical dosage," that is, the prescribed dosage in practice. Unfortunately, with a new drug the setting of such a clinical dosage may be the purpose of the experiment itself; higher and lower dosages must be gradually approached and the expensive experimentation must be prolonged.

Even with these complications and others, not the least of which is that the great majority of drug studies are financed by the drug companies themselves, certain general patterns of findings have begun to emerge.

Sedatives

The drugs most directly related to sleep are the sedatives. These are drugs that cause a general depression of the central nervous system. They are labeled "hypnotics," "depressants," or "sedatives." In general, they "slow down" or "dull" the responsiveness of the central nervous system. Alcohol is by far the most widely used of this group. Among the drugs the barbiturates, or "downers" in street language, are the most frequently prescribed, and they rank high among all drugs prescribed. In 1969, for example, pentobarbital and secobarbital were among the top 20 of the most frequently prescribed drugs in the United States.

The barbiturates are variants of a weak acid—barbituric acid—which was synthesized at the beginning of the twentieth century. Of the some 50 barbiturates marketed today as sedatives, the most prominent are sodium pentobarbital (Nembutal), sodium secobarbital (Seconal), phenobarbital (Eskabarb), and sodium amobarbital (Amytal).

More recently, in the 1950s, an entire new series has been synthesized by the drug companies from a wide range of compounds. This group includes gluethimide (Doriden), methyprylon (Noludar), methaqualone (Quaalude), and flurazepam (Dalmane).

With minor variations, generally in the degree of effect, the influence on sleep of the sedatives is similar. Few differences have been reported among the barbiturates. On the positive side barbiturates, when first taken, reduce the number of awakenings, the amount of wake time after sleep onset, body movements during sleep, and sleep latencies. The latter finding is clouded by the fact that the reduction in latency does not appear to be dose-related. Most of these positive findings have been obtained from mild insomniacs, since little reduction is possible in noninsomniacs who already have very short sleep latencies.

On the negative side certain results have been unequivocally proved. First, all the barbiturates show a marked tolerance effect; higher and higher dose levels are required to maintain the same effect. Second, REM sleep amounts are sharply reduced by initial doses with the effect typically resulting from delays of the initial REM episode and shortened REM amounts in each episode. This reduction in REM amounts may be as high as 60 percent with clinical dosage levels. In the few studies in which the regime has been carried out long enough there is a gradual increase or return of REM. On cessation of the dosage there is a sharp "rebound," or increase in REM amounts compared to the predrug baseline. The data on slow-wave sleep (Stage 4) is more equivocal. In general, the effect seems minimal.

The few studies on chronic users of barbiturates are clear-cut. The most dramatic findings are those associated with REM sleep after withdrawal. This is accompanied by very high "rebound" effects: vivid dreaming, nightmares, and broken or disturbed sleep. Chronic use also results in a reduced level of slow-wave sleep, with a gradual return over several months after withdrawal.

With few exceptions, the other prescriptions act in a similar manner. REM sleep is typically reduced, cessation of the drug results in REM rebound, and there are minimal effects on slow-wave sleep. Chronic usage is associated with disturbed sleep and reduced slow-wave sleep; withdrawal from chronic use typically results in nightmares and even more disturbed sleep.

The effects of alcohol have been studied in some detail. In single doses, the effects on sleep are essentially identical with those described above relative to REM sleep. Slow-wave sleep may increase slightly but will show a reduction on repeated dosages. There is little effect on the reduction of waking time with a mild dosage, but chronic alcohol ingestion is clearly associated with fragmented sleep. On withdrawal of alcohol from chronic dosages there are incidences of nightmares. Indeed, the hallucinations associated with delirium tremens (the "DT's") have been attributed by some workers to a "breakthrough" of REM sleep into the waking state.

The tranquilizers

The tranquilizers are a group of drugs developed to "calm" or "tranquilize" the person in contrast to "sedating" or depressing responsiveness. The tranquilizers are usually divided into the categories of major and minor. The two most widely known of the major tranquilizers are chlorpromazine (Thorazine) and reserpine (Serpasil). These are used to treat the more disturbed behavior for which a person is often hospitalized. The most widely used of the minor tranquilizers are meprobamate (Miltown), chlordiazepoxide (Librium), and diazepam (Valium). These are prescribed in cases of less disturbed behavior for individuals who can generally continue to function in the environment.

The primary use of these drugs is directed toward the control or reduction of behavior disturbances associated with anxiety, tension, and stress rather than toward the production of sleep. However, because these primary disturbances are typically associated with secondary sleep disorders, the interaction with sleep is obvious. In such instances the "sleeping pill" of choice by the physician may be the tranquilizer rather than the sedative.

The effects of these drugs on sleep has been far less widely studied than those of the sedatives. When conducted as clinical studies of problem sleepers the effects have often been compounded by the primary underlying problems of the subjects. The results are quite mixed. In regard to the major tranquilizers (chlorpromazine and reserpine), REM sleep may be increased or decreased and is apparently dosage-related. Slow-wave sleep is increased by chlorpromazine and decreased by reserpine. The amount of waking time during sleep has been reported to be unchanged or increased. The results relative to the minor tranquilizers are also mixed. REM suppression has been associated with meprobamate but not with diazepam or chlordiazepoxide. Slow-wave sleep was generally unaffected by these drugs but waking time was decreased by chlordiazepoxide.

The badly needed studies of the results of chronic usage and withdrawal have not yet been done.

The antidepressants

Even more recent than the tranquilizers in the armamentarium of pharmacology are the "antidepressants." These drugs are directed toward the "euphoriant" side to increase the feelings of well-being and fall into two groups related to their derivative bases: the "trycyclics" and the "monoamine inhibitors." The more prominent of these are two trycyclics: imipramine (Tofanil) and amitriptyline (Elavil), along with the monoamine inhibitor phenelyzine (Nardil).

As with the tranquilizers, the sleep-related studies of these drugs have been limited since the antidepressants are not generally viewed as "sleeping pills" but as aids in the reduction of depression. However, because depression is closely associated with sleep disturbances and the monoamines have been implicated in the biochemistry of sleep, they have received more attention from sleep researchers.

The effects appear to be quite similar to those found in association with the barbiturates: REM sleep is decreased by all three of the drugs cited, with subsequent rebound effect when the drug is withdrawn. Similarly, slow-wave sleep is less markedly affected and the decrease in waking time within sleep presents a mixed picture.

Nonprescription sleeping pills

The nonprescription sleeping pills—Sominex, Sleep-Eze, Nytol, Compos, and Dormin are the most widely known—are widely advertised and sold across the counter without a physician's prescription. Usually the advertisement carefully describes these pills as "helping you get to sleep." The basic ingredient in all the drugs mentioned is methapyraline, which is an antihistamine. Antihistamines were developed primarily to deal with allergic reactions. The effect of these drugs, then, is primarily dependent upon a "side effect" which occurs in varying degrees in individuals with the ingestion of an antihistamine. This is likely to come as a considerable surprise to hay fever victims who may have for years been taking what is actually a sleeping pill for their allergy. The second most prevalent ingredient is scopolomine (or belladona), which is in all the drugs listed except Nytol. Belladona is an ancient drug which is sometimes called the "deadly nightshade" and was used as a poison. Other constituents of these drugs include aspirin, various vitamins, and, in Compos, "passion flower extract."

There have been very few direct laboratory tests of these compounds since most studies have focused on the far more powerful prescription drugs. However, clinical evaluations of the widely used antihistamines, when reporting on them as antihistamines, de-emphasize the "drowsiness" side effects of these drugs and typically report drowsiness as a "possible" consequence. The central nervous system effects of scopolomine have received some attention. Higher dosages result in EEG patterns resembling sleep except that the subjects remain alert and even overreactive.

There have been a few laboratory studies. One analyzed the effects of Sominex on five mildly insomniac subjects. There was no decrease in sleep latency or amount of wake time during sleep. There was evidence of a limited REM suppression. Two further studies have affirmed the likelihood of REM suppression. Two subjects were studied using diphenhydramine (Benadryl), an antihistamine. They showed a 15 percent reduction of REM sleep on the first night of the drug and a 28 percent "rebound" on a drug-free night following three nights of dosage. In a second study, scopolomine was also found to suppress REM. Since both of these drugs appear in Sominex it seems likely that the noted decrease in REM was a real one.

While concerned about the potential REM-suppressor effects of these nonprescription drugs, clinicians concerned with sleep are also concerned about the noneffects of such drugs. They fear that if the expected response is not obtained from the prescribed dosages the person may attempt to solve his problem by increasing the dosage. While the side effects of these pills at the prescribed dosages are likely to be limited, a significant increase may result in worsening the sleep condition. Known side effects include rashes, dizziness, and headaches. Taken in higher dosages there may be deliriums and even death. There is the further concern that such persons may turn toward stronger drugs after experimenting with these medications of limited success but high promise.

The stimulants

Stimulants are intimately implicated in the sleep/wake cycle. In a simple and direct way they are used to suppress or offset sleep. Hard-pressed students, cross-country truck drivers, and people faced with emergencies when continued wakefulness is necessary turn to and find a response from the stimulants. Unfortunately, they may create insomnias or interact with insomnias in a vicious circle. The person may "ride" his stimulant through his pressure period and then, when sleep is possible, find it impossible to "turn off" his stimulant. It continues to oppose sleep and he remains awake. The insomniac is even more liable to enter into the stimulant linkage. Because he is failing to sleep during the night he may feel impelled to offset this lack of sleep (and associated sleepiness) during the demanding day by the use of stimulants. Such an individual faces the following sleep period under a load of stimulants. Then the mild or the chronic insomniac, suffering such poor sleep, may heavily increase his dosage of sedatives or take a heavy dose of sedatives in the early morning hours in a desperate attempt to sleep. As a result he awakens from a heavily drugged sleep, still partially sedated. It is now likely that he will attempt to offset this drugged condition by again turning to stimulants

to achieve even minimal functioning. Maintaining himself through
the day on stimulants, he must face another sleepless night and the
stimulant-sedative-stimulant spiral continues.

The most common of the stimulants is caffeine in coffee, but caffeine
is sometimes taken as a drug in more concentrated form. No-doz is
perhaps the most widely known caffeine-based drug. However, the
most powerful stimulants synthesized during World War II are
amphetamine sulfate (Benzadrine) and methamphetamine pydrochlo-
ride (Methedrine). In the jargon of the street these are the "uppers."

The amphetamines have been widely studied. They do clearly offset
feelings of fatigue and sleepiness. They may accomplish this even in
the face of barbiturate usage or prolonged wakefulness. They act as
expected by increasing latency to sleep, decreasing slow-wave sleep,
and increasing the amount and number of awakenings. In addition,
they significantly reduce the proportion of REM sleep and on
withdrawal from chronic usage show a sharp rebound effect, associated nightmares and sleep disturbances. When used in combination
with barbiturates the effect on REM sleep appears to double and give
a greater effect than either drug alone.

Caffeine has been studied in relatively low dosages—the equivalent
of three to four cups of coffee before retiring. It does show a
disturbance of sleep but the effect is relatively limited: longer
latencies, more awakenings, and evaluations of "poor sleep." There is
little evidence of major effects at this level on the structure of sleep
itself.

Implications

The thin edge between the benefits and potential dangers inherent
in drugs is most clearly exemplified in their relationship to sleep. The
sedatives can hasten sleep and smooth its path. The tranquilizers and
antidepressants can help to calm the agitations and reduce the
depressions that threaten sleep. The stimulants may aid us in offsetting
sleep so that we can carry on during times of critical need. When used
carefully, appropriately, and as temporary expedients they can indeed
serve beneficially our sleep and waking needs in relation to a world
opposing these needs.

However, the effects of these psychoactive drugs should not be
confused with those of the other medicinal drugs. No amount of them
will "cure" the troubled mind or change the pressureful world. When
the direct effect on the nervous system has ceased, the anxieties and
pressures that were there before will not have been ameliorated by the

drug. Unless time, circumstances, or our own efforts have removed the pressures which required the use of the drug, those pressures will continue; they have been only temporarily masked.

Fueled by advertising and the well-meant advice of friends, our beliefs, hopes, and needs for shortcut solutions or "instant grace" may push the problem still further. Although the driving forces behind our insomnia may be beyond the control of drugs, we are likely to try to get the effect we wish by increasing the dosage. If we obtain a little help, more of the same should yield more help. This tendency is compounded by the tolerance aspects of most of the drugs reviewed. With few exceptions, continued use brings about a decreased effectiveness; this phenomenon in turn is quite often responded to by further increasing the dosage.

We are now moving in the direction of abuse and well beyond the range of benefits. Again, whether from their psychological "reinforcing value" or from changes in the central nervous system or from a combination of both, there is an inherent tendency to develop a "dependency" on most of the drugs reviewed. This is particularly true for the sedatives, tranquilizers, and stimulants. The person may begin to take the drug for the sake of its effect and end by taking it from simple need of the drug for its own sake. At this point the person is taking the drug from compulsion and the original cause is a secondary problem.

This move toward abuse may be the course of the drug whether it was prescribed for sleep or for other purposes. However, there are two particular problems associated with drugs and sleep that may exacerbate the unfortunate chain of events: the effects of the drugs on the sleep structure and the potential use of stimulants.

We have seen that the great majority of the drugs reviewed significantly modify the underlying sleep structure, particularly through the suppression of REM sleep. Sleep then becomes a chronic battleground between this suppressor effect and the struggle of the sleep system to maintain its inherent integrity. In this battle, in which neither force can be the winner, sleep becomes fragmented and disturbed. When the drug is stopped there is a "surge" of REM sleep, often accompanied by even more disturbed sleep and nightmares. As a consequence of this pattern of events, the initial sleep problem may become worse and the person may turn to different and larger dosages of drugs. When he tries to stop the upward spiral he is faced with even more disturbed sleep and nightmares and will often revert to drugs simply to go back to the poor, but less disturbed, state of sleep.

Finally, the circle may be completed. Either directly as the result of poor sleep, or as the result of poor sleep compounded by a chronic use of drugs or excessively heavy doses of drugs often taken late at night, the person may feel compelled to turn to stimulants to "get through the day." As we have seen, this can easily lead to a stimulant-sedative-stimulant spiral.

To reiterate: drugs may be useful in the temporary control of sleep; however, the "magic bullet" permitting simple and safe control has not yet been found. Because there are many built-in dangers in the drugs associated with sleep one must proceed with caution.

11

The insomnias

We have now noted a wide range of conditions that may result in disturbed sleep. This chapter is concerned with these troubled states of sleep. When they are sufficiently disturbing and persistent they are appropriately titled "insomnia," from the Latin "nonsleep" (*in* and *somnus*).

Insomnia is a summary term for all real and imagined failures of the sleep process. Almost everyone (a cautious statement) has suffered the occasional presence of sleep disturbance, but for millions it is a chronic problem ranging in its effects from exasperation to desperation.

Insomnias may be chronic or episodic and differ widely in their behavioral manifestations: among these are difficulties in getting to sleep, broken sleep, awakening and being unable to get back to sleep, early awakenings, and combinations thereof. In fact, as we shall see, there are even "insomnias" that show no disturbances of sleep.

The symptoms of insomnia

There are four essential dimensions of insomnia, all of which may be a part of an individual condition: 1) disturbances of sleep as objectively defined, 2) subjective reactions to one's sleep, 3) chronicity or persistence across time of either the objective or subjective reactions, and 4) the severity of the objective or subjective patterns.

THE SLEEP DISTURBANCES OF INSOMNIA

There are three primary sleep disturbances making up the insomniac syndrome: long latencies, awakenings, early termination, and light sleep. They may be singly or simultaneously present and occur with varying degrees of chronicity or severity.

Long latencies: As with all the symptoms this, of course, is a relative phenomenon. How long is long? In sleep laboratories, we typically use a half hour between the time of going to bed and sleep onset as our defining point. We do this because even in the strange surround of the sleep laboratory about 95 percent of all "normal" subjects between the ages of 15 and 50 go to sleep before 30 minutes have passed. Certainly some of the 5 percent are probably demonstrating a form of situational insomnia.

Awakenings: Awakenings take the form of many awakenings, a midsleep gap, or an early awakening. Again, these are relative and are imposed on individual differences in sleep pattern. In an adult population ranging from 20 to 40 years of age we have used more than 30 minutes of wakefulness following the onset of sleep as a conventional definition for amount of wakefulness and five or more awakenings for our definition of number of awakenings. We tend to lower these figures for younger adults and raise these figures for the older group. These "cutoffs" are also derived from laboratory studies and, in general, appear in less than 5 percent of the sleep patterns of "normal subjects" during laboratory sleep.

Early termination: When early terminations do occur they may be simply an extension of a "gap" awakening occurring in the latter part of the night. Again in terms of laboratory studies, by convention a sleep period that terminates spontaneously with less than 360 minutes of sleep (6 hours) is classified in the insomniac pattern.

"Light" sleep: This type of sleep is less certain in its definition and more poorly integrated with subjective complaints about sleep. Subjective complaints about "light" sleep may simply refer to a large number of awakenings or to an early awakening. However, there are two patterns of sleep that are likely to be related to "light" sleep even without awakenings. These are sleep patterns showing very large amounts of Stage 1 sleep and/or reduced Stage 4 sleep. Again, both of these are relative terms and need qualifying. Stage 1 sleep constitutes about 5 percent of laboratory sleep in adults from the age of 20 to 40. Stage 1 sleep exceeding 12 percent is unusually high (less than 5 percent of young adults) with the amount tending to increase with age. Certainly such amounts may well be considered potential disturbances of sleep. Again, "reduced" Stage 4 refers to less Stage 4 than is typical of one's age group. Although this variable has not been validated in its relation to "light" sleep, at least the absence of an expected amount of "deep" sleep holds potential as an indication of a sleep disturbance. By observation of records we would consider less than 5 percent of Stage 4 in a 20- to 30-year-old person or less than 3 percent in a 30- to 40-year-old person potentially symptomatic of an insomniac condition.

SUBJECTIVE COMPLAINTS

The subjective complaints defining insomnia are essentially descriptions of the sleep disturbances described above: difficulties in getting to sleep (long sleep latencies), difficulties in staying asleep (many awakenings, sleep gaps, early awakenings) and light sleep (awakening and, possibly, high amounts of Stage 1 and/or low Stage 4). These, as with the objective disturbances, may be singly or multiply present.

There are several complicating factors relative to the subjective complaints. These complaints may be present although the objective data may show no level of disturbance, or there may be no complaints in the presence of very real objective disturbances. A person with severe complaints may show, on recording of his sleep, a pattern of sleep well within the normal ranges. Conversely, we may find a recorded sleep pattern showing severe disturbance and the person, on questioning, may simply say: "I have no complaints. I guess that's the way the ball bounces."

These discrepancies between objective and subjective aspects of insomnia result in three "types" of insomnias: disturbed sleep with matching subjective complaints, adequate sleep with subjective complaints, and disturbed sleep with no complaints. Naturally, the treatment of these groups must be quite different. One certainly doesn't want to increase the complaints of the disturbed sleeper who has no complaints, nor is the improvement of sleep of the complainant without disturbances very likely.

A primary source of the subjective and objective discrepancies is one's expectancies about sleep. A person who has always slept well may, as a result of aging, be sleeping less well. While having limited disturbances, he may complain bitterly about them. Another individual may have always slept "lightly" and may have adapted to this. Though in fact sleeping "poorly," he may have few complaints.

Some of the exaggerated complaints may represent "projections" of waking-state difficulties on relatively innocent sleep patterns: "I know I could do a better job (win, feel better, feel more secure, be happier, etc.) if I could only sleep better."

How much insomnia?

The range of symptoms associated with insomnia may exist in singular or multiple form. They may be objectively or subjectively present or may be present simultaneously. When this complex picture is compounded by the fact that these symptoms may be chronic or intermittent and exist in varying degrees of severity, it is clear that estimating the extent of insomnia is a difficult task. The problem is further complicated by the fact that one's estimate is clearly dependent upon how and what questions about insomnia are being asked and who is being questioned.

At least three large-scale surveys have included the question "Do you often have trouble falling asleep or staying asleep?" One was a nationwide survey, one involved 1,660 Manhattan residents, and one an urban and rural Puerto Rican population. All yielded the uniform figure of about 14 percent, or one in seven persons sampled, responding yes. In a recent survey of a north Florida county, 1,645 persons randomly selected over the age of 16 years were asked the same question, with possible alternative answers of "never," "sometimes," or "often"; 31 percent answered "sometimes" and again 14 percent answered "often." However, a recent survey conducted of 1,000 households in Los Angeles reported an instance of troubled sleep of 32 percent. In this survey specific symptoms were used to elicit the response: 14 percent reported difficulties in falling asleep; 23 percent reported waking up during sleep; 14 percent reported early awakenings. Thirty-two percent checked at least one category.

Results of shifting both the population and the question can be seen in the response of college students to two questions. When asked "Do you consider yourself an insomniac?" 21 percent responded "sometimes" and $2\frac{1}{2}$ percent responded "always." When asked "Do you have troubled sleep?" 68 percent responded "sometimes" and $2\frac{1}{2}$ percent responded "always."

Age, not surprisingly, sharply affects the degree of "insomnia" expressed. Table 11-1 displays the affirmative responses given by 2,466 individuals in England to four sleep "complaints" in three age groups.

In general, socioeconomic factors such as nationality, racial origin, or income show little or no relationship to insomnia. As expressed by Sir Philip Sidney, "[Sleep is] the indifferent judge between the high

TABLE 11-1 Sleep Complaints in Three Age Groups

	15–25	35–45	55–65
"Less than five hours sleep"	5%	7%	14%
"Longer than an hour and a half to sleep"	2%	4%	14%
"Awaken before five A.M."	1%	3%	10%
"Frequently wake up"	5%	14%	23%

and the low." Surprisingly, however, older and married females show a higher number of complaints in most surveys. In the Los Angeles survey referred to above, females expressed significantly more complaints than males in the total sample and this was even more true for the older female. We call this surprising in the light of our earlier reported laboratory findings indicating that females' sleep patterns show less age change than males'.

How much insomnia then? Certainly repeated figures suggest that sleep is "often" troubled in nearly one person in seven in the general population, and in older persons this is considerably higher. One-half or more of persons questioned have troubled sleep "sometimes."

We have no certain way, however, of estimating the number of individuals for whom insomnia is a desperate battle staged from night to night; a battle that leaves them exhausted and in despair. Again, from indirect evidence the problem appears to be a significantly large one. Each year over $100 million is spent on prescription sedatives. The greater proportion of these sedatives were prescribed by physicians in response to sleep difficulties severe enough to evoke a "call for help." Not included in this grouping are tranquilizers, antidepressants, and alcohol, some of which certainly may be used in coping with sleeplessness, or the nonprescription drugs advertised "to help you get to sleep." Also not included in this description of the extent of the problem are those people fearful of drugs who are struggling with the problem through willpower and rituals.

Sleep clinics

Formal treatment of insomnia as a specific and discrete disorder is quite recent. The first formal sleep clinic was begun in 1963 at the UCLA Medical Center and ten years later there were some half dozen such clinics throughout the country. Prior to this time the complaint of sleeplessness was attended to by a person's physician who, after listening to the complaints, gave one of three typical responses: He reassured the patient and gave him some behavioral routine to follow;

he decided it was an adjunctive symptom of some other disorder and proposed treatment of that disorder or referred the patient to a specialist; he gave the patient a prescriptive drug. Probably the typical response was the latter, with instructions to return if it didn't help.

Sleep clinics do now and in the future will continue to differ from one another in details. However, the common problems are likely to reflect a similarity of approach. In this light, we will outline the general nature of their approach and their treatments. There are three primary differences from earlier, less formal procedures: 1) greater emphasis on the systematic measurement of the symptoms, 2) a more sophisticated diagnosis of the causes based on increased awareness of the multifaceted bases of insomnia, and 3) the different and more cautious approach to the use of drugs in treatment.

In regard to the presenting symptoms, the basic problem lies in the not-infrequent discrepancy between the subjective evaluation by the patient and the objective presence of sleep disturbances. This matter can be readily differentiated by the use of the EEG as an objective definition of sleep disturbances.

A report from the Stanford Sleep Clinic emphasizes this problem and also provides an excellent picture of the objective character of sleep disturbances in patients who voluntarily seek help for their problem. Table 11-2 presents the sleep parameters of 55 individuals complaining of severe, chronic insomnia who had been recorded by the EEG for 3 consecutive nights and were receiving either no medication or an inactive placebo. There were 26 females (average age 50 years; age range 32–68) and 29 males (average age 43 years; age range 19–68). The table reports the second night of recording.

TABLE 11-2 Selected Sleep Parameters of 55 Insomniacs (minutes)

	Latency	Wake After Sleep Onset	Total Sleep Time
Average	30.3	49.5	379.5
Range	1.5–421.6	2.0–287.7	160.1–566.5

While clearly different from a population of good sleepers and showing a general picture of disturbed sleep, the range within the population was very large. Individual characteristics and the complex of insomnia symptoms are even more revealing. The authors of the study applied specific insomnia criteria to each patient: 30-minute onset latency, wake time of more than 30 minutes after sleep onset, and less than 6½ hours of total sleep. On the second night only 12 individuals (21 percent) met the sleep-latency criteria, 26 (46 percent) the wake time-after-onset criteria, and 30 (54 percent) the sleep-time criteria. Only 2 met all three criteria and 12 met none of them. On the third night 13 individuals (23 percent) met the sleep-latency criteria, 25 (45 percent) the wake time-after-onset criteria, and 31 (55 percent) the total sleep criteria. Only 3 met all three criteria and 10 met none of them. Unfortunately the report does not indicate which did or did not meet the criteria across the 2 nights.

The treatment of insomnia

We've seen that the symptoms of insomnia are widely diverse in objective and subjective patterns and degree of chronicity and severity. In the preceding chapters we have discussed a wide range of conditions and circumstances that may disrupt sleep: aging, situation, pathology, anomalies of sleep and drugs. Within these complexities, the treatment of insomnia follows the pattern of the treatment of any disorder: that is, it begins with a careful description of the problem and a search for the cause.

While the EEG must ultimately be used to define the specific pattern of the sleep disturbance, we usually begin with the case history. What precisely is the problem with sleep? Is there trouble getting to sleep? Is there trouble staying asleep? Are there awakenings from sleep? How many? When? Is there too little sleep? Is there too much sleep? Is there sleep during the day? When did this change begin? Were there particular circumstances? Are there some reasons that you can think of for not being able to sleep? What have you done about it? Have you used drugs? What kind? How long?

Let us assume that the therapist is either a physician or a psychologist working in collaboration with a physician. As a result of the case history, several alternatives may be followed.

The therapist may decide that the symptomatology is not sufficiently clear and the patient is asked to keep a sleep log for a week or more and to return with it. Alternatively, the person may be asked to sleep one or more nights in the laboratory or the clinic so that sleep recordings may be obtained. However, the symptomatology may be sufficiently clear from the case history to give strong indications of the probable cause. In such cases the EEG may be considered unnecessary to begin treatment or to warrant referral of the person.

The treatment itself will differ in relation to the inferred etiology, or cause. Generally, these will fall into six categories, which we will discuss with frequent reference to the earlier chapters. The categories are situational, benign, rhythmic, sleep anomalies, secondary sleep disorders and drugs.

SITUATIONAL INSOMNIAS

The primary clues to these insomnias for the therapist are recent onset and/or limited sleep disturbances. The situational insomnias are those brought about by self-imposed or externally imposed circumstances which cause the person to continue responding to the waking world. He tries to go to sleep or to continue sleeping, but he is also still attempting to cope with the world. As we discussed in Chapter 6, so long as these tendencies are strong, the chances of effective sleep are reduced. The causes and circumstances for such behavior are manifold: new business opportunity or problems; new developments in a love relationship, either a beginning or an end; a death of a near one; a critical life decision; a strong guilt about one's recent behavior; an abysmal failure. These are a few of many examples. All have in common strong involvement of the individual.

The response of the therapist is first to point up the naturalness of the sleep problem. He will, in addition, consider prescribing a carefully controlled use of either sedatives or drugs with safeguards or follow-up and a caution about their use. He is very likely to point to the problem and assert that until the problem is reduced the disturbance will be there.

Sometimes it is apparent that the situation is likely to be a chronic one. In such circumstances the therapist's only alternative is to advise the person about the probable cause and make suggestions for changing the circumstances. A particularly interesting case was reported by Dr. Peter Hauri. A young man reported being unable to sleep. He was at the time going to school and sleeping in his mother's house. Dr. Hauri asked the young man when he had last been able to sleep well. The young man replied that it had been during an arduous mountain climb when he and several companions were trapped on a rock face by a sudden snowstorm, tied together for the night. In these difficult circumstances he had slept well. Dr. Hauri suggested that he consider moving away from home!

BENIGN INSOMNIAS

Benign disturbances are those in which the person reports poor sleep but the limits or problems with sleep are well within the range of normal sleep. In short, the person's sleep is falling short of his expectancies. Three frequent sources of these complaints are the aged, natural short sleepers, or individuals who are in circumstances that are likely to cause sleep disruption but are likely to change.

We have seen in Chapter 4 that sleep often becomes less adequate as a natural part of aging and these changes, as they contrast with the previously undisturbed sleep, may result in the person thinking something is wrong with him. Most often the therapist will obtain an EEG. If he determines that this sleep pattern is well within the range of age changes and can find no other circumstances in the case, he is likely to advise the person about the age changes and attempt to reassure him.

Sometimes an individual will report failing to "get enough sleep" or being unable to "get to sleep" and these problems may be merely reflecting his own natural pattern of sleep. He is a natural "short" sleeper (Chapter 7) and he is trying to be what he considers a "normal" sleeper. In these circumstances the therapist is likely to ask the subject to keep a careful sleep log for several weeks. After making certain that there are no other problems involved, he is again likely to reassure the patient, suggest to him that he may be fortunate rather than unfortunate, and urge him to use his extra time of wakefulness effectively.

A contrasting case is that of the "long" sleeper who is getting inadequate sleep and awakening groggy or feeling sleepy during the day as a result of trying to match his sleep time to some mythical norm or perhaps his spouse's sleep. Again, reassurance and adjustment of sleep amount are the best prescriptions.

Not infrequently, the "situational" insomnia may be viewed as natural or benign and the therapist will avoid treatment. The person under some situational stress is very likely to focus much of his attention on his sleep disturbances: "If I could only get enough sleep I could cope better" or "Things wouldn't be so bad if I could only get enough sleep." The therapist's role is, again, to reassure the patient that the disturbed sleep is natural and probably not a major contributor to the problem at hand.

It is important to note that in the benign insomnias the therapist makes every effort to avoid treatment. Treatment is judged to be either not possible (in cases due to aging or natural limited sleep) or not necessary (in temporary disturbing situations). In these instances the therapist's role is one of reassurance. In all cases, however, he must perform a careful follow-up to confirm his judgment.

Arrhythmic insomnias

The arrhythmic insomnias could readily be named the "Edison" effect. The creation of the electric light yielded the easy potential of selecting one's behavior across the 24 hours. Our sleep is no longer regularized by the setting and rising of the sun or at least by the inconvenience of poor and expensive lighting. As a consequence, our sleep time is determined by choice and this choice follows our interests and needs, in contrast to our rhythms. Not only do we simply vary our sleep onset time in terms of several hours around an average, but we may shift it radically and for varying periods of time such as under shift-work conditions.

As a consequence of shifting sleep times, the rhythmic cues for going to sleep or staying asleep are reduced or even eliminated. The effects of the disruptions of rhythms of sleep were discussed in Chapter 5 on the effects of time variation. To reiterate, when sleep-onset time is highly variable the body simply doesn't know what is expected of it and the support of "going-to-sleep" bodily cues is reduced or lost. The onset of sleep becomes less likely. When there are attempts to sleep at a time when one is typically awake, sleep is characterized by a changed rhythm and more frequent and early awakenings.

The arrhythmic insomnias are seldom severe enough to result in sleep clinic visits. However, insomniacs of all types are frequently arrhythmic and this imposition on their already fragile sleep systems may be exaggerating their disorder. Further, a solid rhythm will often help treatment. As a consequence, a program of regularizing sleep is a typical part of the treatment of most insomnia. Indeed, it is often reported that merely keeping a record of one's sleep for several weeks has resulted in "cures."

Sleep anomalies

We have discussed the sleep anomalies or primary sleep disorders associated with the sleep mechanisms in Chapter 8. The critical cues in these cases are the intrusions of sleep into the waking process (narcolepsy and hypersomnia) or the presence of wakelike behaviors within sleep (sleepwalking, night terrors, nightmares, and enuresis). These are typically detected by means of the case history but effective and certain diagnosis will often require EEG studies.

The sleep-intrusive conditions of narcolepsy and hypersomnia, appearing as they do within the waking state, frequently interfere with day-to-day adjustments, making their treatment essential. It is critical in both instances to make accurate diagnoses. There must be a careful distinction between a simple feeling that one needs a lot of sleep, or a cumulated need for sleep in the daytime that may result from poor sleep habits or insomnia, and the compelling, excessive sleep response associated with true narcolepsy and hypersomnia. Further, one must avoid mistaking the hypersomnias that may arise from some underlying neuropathology. Sleep research is increasingly clarifying the nature of these disorders, and diagnosis and treatment is possible with increasing confidence in sleep clinics.

The wake-intrusive disturbances of sleep seen in sleepwalking, night terrors, nightmares, and enuresis are all age-related and typically involve cases in early childhood. Because these are often naturally occurring aspects of development, the treatment may frequently involve simply reassurance of parents and giving advice on how to react to and handle the events. The therapist must, of course, determine whether these disturbances are of unusual severity or signal other underlying problems. In the former instance the sleep clinic will undertake the management of the disorder and in the latter a referral may be indicated.

Occasionally, the wake-intrusive disturbances extend into adulthood; when they are frequent and disturbing, treatment must be undertaken.

In all instances of the sleep anomalies an important aspect of treatment is an emphasis on the fact that they are "extensions" of sleep itself. Focus is on the treatment of the sleep disturbances rather than on some more awesome or complicated "mental" problem. A reassurance that the sufferer is not "mentally sick" but has an understandable deviation in the way that he is sleeping is often a great relief.

SECONDARY SLEEP DISORDERS

It was noted that many primary pathological conditions result in disturbed sleep. These sleep disturbances may be an early or more obvious aspect of the underlying primary problem and the person may seek help in dealing with this secondary symptom.

We discussed the primary dysfunctions under the categories of neuropathologies, physiopathologies, and psychopathologies. The primary conditions often require specialized skills in diagnosis and treatment. It is a usual procedure for sleep clinics to require or undertake a general physical examination as a part of the routine. If a primary disorder is noted in this examination a referral for speciality diagnosis and treatment generally follows. Further, the therapists in sleep clinics are particularly sensitive to those pathologies which have sleep as a part of their symptomatology. If during treatment a suspicion arises that there might be an underlying pathology, referral for a more specialized diagnosis is likely. The sleep clinic in this process may run an EEG recording of the sleep of the patient before referral and will typically provide comments on the associated sleep problem for the physician to whom the patient is referred.

In some instances of primary disorders the diagnostic and treatment skills required may be available within the sleep clinic or within the capabilities of the physician approached for treatment. This is particularly true in the cases of psychopathology, since sleep clinics are often operated within departments of psychiatry in medical schools and the individual approached for help may be a psychiatrist or psychologist. In these circumstances, treatment is directly undertaken with the judicious use of drugs and psychotherapy.

Drug-related insomnias

We have seen in our earlier chapter on drugs that most of the psychoactive drugs result in REM suppression. The chronic usage of such drugs is typically associated with a badly disturbed sleep pattern characterized particularly by frequent awakenings. We described the sleep world resulting from the chronic suppression of REM sleep as a "battleground" with sleep itself often being the victim. Because of this and because drug dependency, which may or may not have been associated with insomnia at its outset, is not an uncommon event on today's scene, insomnias resulting from drug abuse are by no means uncommon.

In writing about his sleep clinic experiences, a leading sleep researcher said: "Whenever a patient complains of insomnia and gives a history of taking sleeping pills, our tentative diagnosis is always hypnotic dependency or drug-dependency insomnia." He goes on to vividly describe the classical course of these insomnias:

> If you take a normal subject and give him 200 milligrams of a barbiturate at bedtime, his sleep time will increase. REM time will be reduced. If we give the same dose every night at bedtime, very quickly, within a week or two, the increase in sleep time will disappear and, indeed, the total sleep time may actually be less than the base line value, even though the patient is taking a barbiturate every night. At

this point, the dose can be increased and the same cycle of events will be repeated. As the subject takes more and more barbiturates, he becomes more and more dependent. . . . Thus a normal subject can be converted into a patient who, although he may be taking thousands of milligrams of barbiturate every night, nonetheless has insomnia. With one or two exceptions, all sleeping pills will always cause or worsen insomnia. . . . The all-night sleep patterns of patients who are taking large doses of barbiturates show no stage 3 and 4, very little REM sleep, many arousals, and some reduction in sleep time. (William Dement and J. Villablanca, "Clinical Disorders in Man and Animal Model Experiments," in *Basic Sleep Mechanisms*, eds. Olga Petre-Quadens and J. Schlag [New York: Academic Press, 1974], p. 323.)

To this description of the route of the barbiturate user must be added the similar patterns previously noted in regard to other sedatives such as alcohol, many of the tranquilizers and antidepressants, and the stimulants. The extent of the problem is related, of course, to extent of the drug involvement in terms of chronicity and the amount of the drugs being taken.

Obviously the treatment of these dependency insomnias involves, as a first step, the withdrawal of the drug causing the disturbance. Here there is an immediate complication, which has been identified as "Drug withdrawal insomnia." With abrupt withdrawal there are frequently physical withdrawal syndromes resulting from the drug abstinence itself and which minimally involve "jitters" and nervousness. These conditions, when compounded by apprehensiveness about "getting along" without the drug, result in difficulty getting to sleep. After getting to sleep, as we have seen in cases when REM-suppressor drugs are withdrawn, there is a sharp REM "rebound," accompanied by highly fragmented and disrupted sleep with frequent vivid and horrid dreams. Outside of the therapeutic situation these effects are often so disturbing that the person voluntarily trying to stop taking drugs may be driven back to his "poor but anything is better than this" sleep and into continued or increasing dosages.

If the problem is essentially confined to sleep disturbance the treatment is typically one of very gradual withdrawal of the drug. This course of withdrawal is determined by the level of drug dosages that the patient has been following. The element of gradualness is emphasized by the recommendation of one of the most sophisticated clinicians in this area for "one therapeutic dose every five days." When it is recognized that many patients have boosted their intake well beyond a single therapeutic dose per day, the recommended withdrawal regime is indeed gradual—taking weeks or months to accomplish.

This withdrawal is accompanied by an investigation into withdrawal effects, particularly the possibilities of "drug withdrawal insomnia." There is a continued search for the basis of the original insomnia. In addition, there are recommendations of physical and timing regimens to aid better sleep.

In some instances, of course, the insomnias presented are secondary symptoms of a drug "addiction" or dependency per se. In such cases, like the treatment of the secondary sleep disorders described above, the problem is the treatment of the primary disorder—in this case drug dependency—which will probably require referral or specialized treatment as such. Chronic alcoholism would be such an example. The special treatment, however, should take into account the certain and associated problems of sleep—particularly those occurring during the "withdrawal" period.

ENDOGENOUS INSOMNIAS

Some as yet unknown but probably small number of insomnias may be the direct result of a failure of the underlying sleep/waking mechanism itself. A particularly striking example of this was recently reported in Lyon, France. A person reported to a neurological clinic with the primary complaint of muscular twitching. On questioning he reported an inability to sleep. This was quickly verified by EEG recordings. During five nights of recording, the total sleep time per night averaged only 26 minutes almost exclusively comprised of Stage 1 sleep. The recordings were extended to 24-hour recordings and sleep was not occurring during the day. A wide variety of drugs proved totally ineffective. However, treatment with massive doses of a drug directly related to brain serotonin levels resulted in sleep periods of up to 4 or 5 hours with a return of the sleep stages.

This, of course, is a rare example but we know that the sleep mechanism is a complex neurological and biochemical system. We must believe that in some insomnias the system can be uniquely "off." It can only be hoped that future research in the biochemistry of sleep and careful attention to the insomnias of unspecifiable causes will both elucidate and control these insomnias.

Implications

Sleep does not flow smoothly in the stream of life for a considerable number of people. Surveys repeatedly cite about 14 percent of the population—or one person in seven—having frequent "difficulties" with their sleep.

These difficulties take a variety of forms but their basic syndrome includes difficulties in getting to sleep or staying asleep. The picture is complicated by the degree and chronicity of the difficulties and the frequent lack of linkage between subjective and objective disturbance.

Insomnias result from a variety of causes. Some, the secondary sleep disorders, stem from primary pathological conditions—illnesses. Some, such as narcolepsy, night terrors, and the like, are primary dysfunctions of the sleep process itself. We may include here the breakdowns of the sleep process with aging and the probable presence of endogenous insomnias. The secondary sleep disorders require treatment of the primary conditions with special attention given to the associated sleep disturbances. The primary sleep disorders require focus on the underlying sleep process with much emphasis on the understanding of the disorder as a sleep disorder in and of itself.

A significant proportion of the insomnias, however, are created by our environment and our own behavior. In this sense, it is possible to argue that many insomnias are modern; exacerbated if not created by "our times." We have discussed these under the situational, benign, arrhythmic, and drug-related insomnias and the "stress" reactions of the psychoneuroses. Treatment of each of these involves a person giving up a particular behavior pattern or set of beliefs.

We cannot argue that in the past there were no situations that "pressed" into and on sleep, that there were no neuroses or self-conflicts and doubts, or that individuals did not overevaluate their sleep disturbances. It does seem, however, that modern times have created more need and opportunity for such circumstances to exist.

Certainly a strong case can be made for the modernity of the drug-related and arrhythmic insomnias. While sleep potions have been sought and used throughout history, the modern era of "sleeping pills" and associated tranquilizers, antidepressants, and stimulants is unprecedented. When this volume is compounded with the particularized potential effects on sleep, the past pales and references to a modern insomnia seem appropriate.

We have noted that the arrhythmic insomnias resulting from irregular or displaced sleep times may well be called the "Edison" effect. Because of the electric light we may and do prolong the day or even change night into day. As a result, sleep may be unhinged from its underlying rhythmic character and lose an element of its stability. Certainly some individuals in the past "burned the midnight oil," but many more today violate nature's clock.

Insomnias are signs of a natural and inherently well-ordered response under stress. They are clues speaking with a bodily wisdom to us about ourselves and the world we are living in. We should not overreact to them with blame or fear, or use them as excuses. We should not ignore them either. At the least we can try to understand what they are signaling. Often they are a price we must pay to live as we do. Often we can respond to them by changing our beliefs or behaviors. If the insomnia and/or the problem it is signaling is in the extreme we can seek the help which, each year and each day, is increasingly effective.

12

Sleep and performance

Some readers have probably been experiencing a growing impatience. This is very likely true of those who are natural pragmatists or who cut their teeth in the early 1970s on the rattler of "relevance." A description of the nature of and the variations in sleep is not sufficient. Their most natural question is: "So sleep varies . . . does it make any difference? If we sleep differently, poorly, or not at all, what difference does it make in our waking world?"

In the jargon of the experimenter, we have primarily considered sleep as a *dependent* variable, that is, as a response modified by, changed by, or "dependent" upon changes in other factors: for example, age, prior wakefulness, or drugs. However, sleep can be viewed as an *independent* variable, that is, as a factor determining or modifying other responses. In this chapter we will look at variations in sleep as these variations are related to other behaviors. Specifically, we shall try to answer the appropriately raised question of the pragmatist: What differences do differences in sleep make?

Some problems of measurement

To find the effect of one thing on another the general procedure is simple enough; you vary (or find naturally occurring variations in) the "influencer" and find out whether there is an effect. In our question at hand, you vary sleep and find out what happens. As you look more closely at the problem, however, it almost immediately becomes more complicated.

First, consider the matter of varying sleep. There are two obvious questions: What kind of variations are we talking about and how much variation? No sleep at all for a day, two days or more? Less sleep for one night or for many nights? Different kinds of sleep—for example, reduced or no REM sleep, or "poor" sleep? All of these seem reasonable questions as all these elements do occur and possibly have real but differing effects. We will consider each of these variations separately under sections of total deprivation of sleep (no sleep), partial deprivation of sleep (less sleep), selective deprivation (limited kinds of sleep).

The problems of measuring the consequences are yet more complex: what do we measure and to what do we attribute the effects if they are present? The specific behaviors that may be affected are almost limitless: from eye blinks to performances in marathons, from higher responsiveness to pain to less exalted thoughts. Which of these should we measure? Even attempts to sort these into more fundamental dimensions are fraught with difficulties. Reaction time? Motor efficiency? Perceptual scanning? Attention? Problem solving? Memory? Endurance? Within even these broader choices the strings of subcategories are awesome. For example, reaction time: With or without forewarning? Complex or simple signals? Visual or auditory signals? High or low energy signals? Motor versus sensory sets?

Having made a choice and a measurement there remains an awesome difficulty. Performance is a mélange of three complex variables: capacity, motivation, and adaptive compensation. Performance may be degraded but was it due to an inability to perform or an unwillingness to perform? Or suppose there is no change? Was he less capable but "compensated" by trying harder or using more energy, and at what expense?

There are no pat answers to the problems of measuring performance. Guided sometimes by guess, sometimes by practical interests, sometimes by theory or previous work, researchers have tried. Their attempts are what we shall report on.

Underlying the problems we have cited is a particularly plaguing one for sleep researchers: control. We have stated that the general procedure involves modifying the variable in question and measuring the effect. We can be sure that the effect found is due to the condition varied only if it and no other condition was varied. In a well-controlled laboratory experiment we hold everything constant except the critical variable. During sleep deprivation, however, the subject is not just "not sleeping." He knows he is not sleeping. He uses up more energy than he would if he were asleep. He receives totally different stimulation. Most important, he thinks or "expects" that the loss of sleep will have some effects. Are the consequences obtained a function of the absence of sleep or due to the presence of these and other "uncontrolled variables"? A particularly good example of this problem is seen in studies that use animals. They at least do not know that your purpose is for them to stay awake. Their natural response to prolonged wakefulness is to sleep and they must be "instructed" to stay awake. Since the need to sleep is quite strong (and gets stronger with the passage of time) the animal has to be put under a severe regime of "punishment" for sleeping. Whatever its behavior—which is, for example, often quite aggressive—was it due to the stress and punishment rather than simply the lack of sleep?

These complexities have not been introduced to seek pity for the poor sleep researcher—although a bit of tolerance would not be amiss—rather they are cautionary statements. They will, I hope, serve to make us cautious about generalizations about the effects of sleep and performance in "real life"—whether from our own experiences, our guesses, or the reports or guesses of others. When I see a bleary-eyed colleague say, "I feel lousy. I didn't get enough sleep last night," I am prone to ask, "What did you do instead?" When a student tells me that he kept falling asleep and couldn't study at 4:00 A.M. I tend to add, "You probably wouldn't have wanted to study that material at four P.M. when studying would have been even easier."

I hope that the preceding description of these complications will help to justify my almost exclusive dependence on laboratory studies. At least in these studies every effort has been made to minimize the problems we have raised. Sleep has varied in degree and kind, a wide variety of performances have been carefully assessed, and as much care as possible has been taken with controlling extraneous factors.

Finally, let the stated complexities serve as a good warning background for any generalizations made. Because we are far from certain of consequences in this area, what will be said must be grounded very much on judgment rather than on fully substantiated and certain facts.

Total sleep deprivation

The search for the consequences of total sleep loss has been a long one; the first animal study was performed in 1894 and the first human study in 1896. However, in spite of the critical problem involved, the effort has not been intensive. A very complete 1963 literature review showed that 37 animal experiments had been performed in the 69 years, 18 of these in one laboratory. Two subsequent experiments have been reported from our laboratories. Into the 1940s, nearly 50 years of research had yielded only 16 human sleep deprivation experiments exceeding a one-night sleep loss; these involved a total of 49 subjects. In the following 30 years there have been about 20 total-sleep-deprivation experiments.

One possible explanation of this rather limited body of data is that the results were thought to be so obvious and striking that there seemed little need for repetition. As we shall see, this is hardly the case. In fact, our review would suggest just the contrary. It is more likely that because the results have been so contradictory or the striking findings so few, research has been discouraged.

Let us first consider the animal data. Not unexpectedly, the majority of these experiments have concentrated on physiological rather than behavioral consequences. They began dramatically. The initial experiment conducted in Italy in 1894 found that puppies died after 4–6 days without sleep. They showed a sharp drop in their temperature (from 7–9 degrees Fahrenheit), a decrease in their red blood count, and changes in their brain matter. Repeating the experiment three years later another Italian investigator, using adult dogs, found death occurring after 9–17 days and a drop in temperature. However, there was no decrease in the red blood count and completely different brain changes were found. In a subsequent series of experiments in the early 1900s with larger numbers of dogs, a French investigator, using deprivation periods of up to 21 days, found no changes in blood characteristics, blood pressure, heart rate, respiration, or body temperature. He found yet another set of brain changes. Kleitman in 1927 studied 12 puppies and their litter mates, who were not deprived of sleep. The puppies were kept awake from 2 to 7 days. There were no changes in body temperature, heart rate, respiration, blood sugar, or white cell count. He did confirm the earlier finding of a drop in red blood cell count. Neurological examinations of the brains were entirely negative.

A careful review of the physiological consequences of prolonged deprivation in animals reveals few clearly documented and consistent changes that could be ascribed to sleep loss. The typical substantial weight loss, the total disruption of the biorhythms underlying the physiological processes, and the stress required to maintain wakefulness could easily account for any effects that have been noted.

Several behavioral findings are startling. First, animals have been kept awake for extremely long periods of time and, within such experiments, there was a wide range of individual differences in response. In the French experiment noted earlier, dogs were kept awake "in no case beyond the point of extreme sleepiness." The range of sleep deprivation was from 30 hours to 505 hours—or 21 days! In an experiment with rabbits kept awake in a slowly rotating cage that required a change in position every 7½ seconds, "extreme sleepiness" occurred between 6 and 31 days. In an experiment in our laboratory 12 young rats were placed on a slowly rotating wheel surrounded by water. Only one animal failed to maintain his wakefulness over 27 days and this failure occurred after 16 days of no sleep.

A common behavioral consequence has been hyperirritability or aggressiveness. This appears after a considerable period of time under the imposed regimes. In the 27-day experiment with rats immediate and sustained aggressiveness when two sleep-deprived animals were paired with each other began after 16 days.

Extreme sleepiness is, of course, present. In rats this manifests itself in an almost immediate "burst" of sleep in the absence of stimulation and, in dogs, in a general decreased responsiveness to the surround.

An example of the continual and often ingenious battle for sleep was seen in one of our rats. He managed to climb to the top of his chamber, up smooth steel walls, and hook his teeth into a meshed wire covering the chamber. There he was found sleeping while suspended by his teeth!

The method of deprivation makes a marked difference. In one experiment in our laboratory we maintained wakefulness under two regimes; one group of rats was shocked immediately on showing any signs of sleep, while the other group was stimulated positively by walking, handling, feeding, and constant nonpunitive stimulation. The shocked group, after from 18–30 hours, could not be kept awake by almost continuous shock; immediately after the shock they would show sleep signs. The other group continued to be alert, ate well, and showed few signs of extreme sleepiness after 4 days of wakefulness.

One final provocative finding occurred in a replicated experiment. Using a water maze that required the learning of a complex pattern in order to escape quickly, rats deprived of sleep for 24–48 hours performed from 10–20 percent better than a matched nondeprived group of animals.

Although many of us have stayed up all night and some of us longer, such occasions were most often under unusual circumstances and frequently involved "catnaps" and going to sleep as quickly as we could. Let us begin, then, with a general description of what people are like when the matter is just one of keeping awake.

We recently completed an experiment which, in the planning, we were not sure that we could carry out. Subjects were required to stay awake from 8:00 A.M. of the first day, through two nights without sleep, until 11:00 P.M. of the third day on two widely separated occasions. They were awake continuously for 51 hours. The difficult problem was that on one of these occasions they were to lie in bed during the time when they would usually have been asleep (11:00 P.M.–7:00 A.M.) *but* they had to remain awake. On the other occasion they were kept active during the "sleep period" by regular sessions on an exercise bicycle. We were trying to separate out the effects of energy loss during sleep deprivation from the loss of sleep itself. We were not sure that we could keep the bed-rest subjects awake.

There were as many individual reactions as there were subjects, in the area of detailed responses, but a number of features were common to all and we shall describe these general reactions.

First, the exercise condition was preferred by all subjects. All of the difficulties associated with staying awake were markedly compounded by having to lie in bed.

The first night passed easily and if there was sleepiness it came between four and six in the morning. However, the subjects could easily "hyp" themselves up to override any such tendencies. During the first day there were few complaints about or evidence of sleepiness; the subjects cheerfully performed their tasks and, in between, played checkers, chess, and card games in high spirits. The whole experiment was viewed as a kind of game.

During the second night without sleep, moods began to change markedly. This was particularly true of the bed-rest time. Staying awake became a struggle. If the experimenter left the bed-rest room, even briefly, EEG signs of sleep would occur (the subjects were being continuously monitored on the EEG). When the experimenter would call to the subjects or, often, be required to shake them awake, they would usually deny that they had been asleep. Tempers often flared. The exercise periods were actually looked forward to since they helped to offset sleep tendencies. The sleep pressures, as on the first day, occurred most strongly during the early-morning hours, when sleep became almost overpowering.

During the following day the subjects, though trying hard, would almost inevitably fall asleep during a half-hour task of monitoring a tone signal and have to be awakened. They were no longer cheerful and were not interested in their games. The mood was generally one of seriousness, even grimness. Spontaneity was missing and they did what they were told to do apathetically. They moved around the laboratory listlessly and, in the absence of stimulation, would lapse into sleep while most often vigorously denying that they had done so.

We saw no really "strange" behavior. Attention wandered, there were grumbles, and certainly there was little liveliness, but the subjects were simply "flattened" people doing a dull job in a dulled way.

I have observed longer deprivations and read the literature

carefully. The pattern of our experiment is extended. Inactivity results in immediate sleep and these tendencies are overwhelming in the early-morning hours. However, when engaged in some short-term, intensive effort, the person seems able to "come out of it." The problems center around straying attention and irritation at having to fight sleep. The usual physical complaints are about "itchy" eyes or "feeling tired" and, in the third and fourth days, of "double" vision and "feeling unreal." After about the fourth day this picture is stabilized with little change. The person is as sleepy as possible but continues to function.

Before turning our attention to behavior and performance changes let us quickly review the physiological findings associated with prolonged sleep loss. These fall into three general categories: neurological, physiological, and biochemical.

Neurologically, four consistent findings have resulted from general neurological tests on sleep-deprived persons: a fine hand tremor, a difficulty in focusing the eyes (diplopia), a drooping of the eyelids, and an increased sensitivity to pain. A wide variety of other neurological tests—on various reflexes, sensation, and on orientation—have shown no decrement. Specific and repeated findings associated with the EEG have been noted and replicated. As early as 1937 a progressive reduction in alpha-type brainwave activity was found. This has been recently confirmed by an intensive study of four subjects undergoing nine days of sleep loss. In this experiment, a significant "recovery" of alpha occurred after the five days of sleep loss but it remained well below the nondeprived level. There are arguments among researchers as to whether this "lost" alpha reflects a moving toward Stage 1 sleep or is the result of extra concentration and effort by subjects to offset sleepiness (see Chapter 2).

Studies of physiology and the autonomic nervous system in relation to sleep loss have been remarkable in their repeated findings of no change. This has been true for body weight, heart rate, respiration, and blood pressure. After five days (but not before) emotional response measures such as those used in lie detector tests (skin resistance, heart rate, respiration changes) begin to show a sluggishness.

Body temperature has shown consistent but puzzling effects. All studies have confirmed an overall decrease in body temperature while still retaining the pattern associated with the person's usual sleep/waking rhythm. It continues to rise during the person's regular waking period and to fall during the usual sleep period. However, a study of prolonged deprivation beyond five days showed a tendency for temperature levels to rise after that time and by the ninth day to reach baseline levels.

Blood samples and urine samples after prolonged deprivation have been carefully assayed for signs of biochemical changes. The results have been generally inconsistent and remarkably limited. As described by one of the more sophisticated investigators when questioned about the biochemical changes observed at 205 hours of sleep loss they were said to be "modest, subtle, and slight." This is in spite of prolonged sleep loss, disrupted biorhythms, additional energy expenditures, and possibly altered dietary habits.

But what of behavioral changes? Before we look at specific test performance let us look at the way sleep-deprived subjects are behaving. There is very little doubt that some "crazy" behavior has been reported. The critical questions are how much, what kind, and why. The first is easy to answer: very little. The second is a little more difficult. The more typical "strange" behaviors are transient lapses into disassociated thoughts or visual hallucinations. The third question is an even more difficult one since the source of any behavior is probably multiple in causation.

If we confine our definition of "crazy" behavior to gross, highly disturbed behavior which the person needs help in controlling, we have some solid statistics. First, such behavior has not been reported in sleep losses of less than some 60 hours, or two and a half days. In one study of 350 soldiers who went 112 hours without sleep, 7 of them showed temporary disturbed "psychotic"-type behavior and this occurred in the third day in all instances. In a study performed in Czechoslovakia only 2 subjects out of 26 showed a "disturbed" response in 126 hours of deprivation. This occurred in these subjects after 60 and 72 hours respectively.

The most typical of the extreme behaviors have taken the form of delusions about the experiment. For example, the subject may assert that the experimenters are attempting to fool him. There may be brief, hallucinatory responses. These latter are usually visual or tactile, in contrast to the more typical auditory hallucinations of the psychotic patient. For example, the subject may feel that he has cobwebs on his face.

If one "counts" momentary confusions, losses of one's train of thought, bursts of irritation, feeling "spacy," or general apathy—in short, exaggerations of our daily behavior—there are frequent instances of such "unusual" behavior after about three days of sleep loss. The most frequent behavior changes are transient inattentions, confusions, or misperceptions. While reciting the alphabet a subject may suddenly interject a comment about his wife or, during a conversation, lose his train of thought completely. Not infrequently, in experiments involving a group of subjects, the group will become "overresponsive" to a problem. They may all decide that the food has become markedly worse and their individual responses to it will become exaggerated.

Where does this behavior come from? Most of the extreme florid behavior has been traceable to predeprivation "chinks" in the individual personality structure. One of the best reported examples is a vivid hallucinatory response which occurred after 168 hours. This was described as follows in a report:

> At 168 hours of sleeplessness, R.S. suddenly went "berserk" during the psychomotor tracking task. He screamed in terror and pulled his electrodes off and fell to the floor sobbing and muttering incoherently about a gorilla and repeatedly asking to be taken off the experiment. Luckily, one of the investigators (E.J.K.) was present and was impressed that R.S. was behaving like a child who was having a night terror. He asked R.S. if his reaction was anything like any of his previous experiences including night terrors when he was a little boy. R.S. confirmed this and talked with much effect about his night terrors when he was 5 or 6 years old. These consisted of seeing Humpty Dumpty, "like in the picture books," being harassed by a gorilla. He then went on to relate that as he was tracking on the oscilloscope screen, it gradually changed and became Humpty Dumpty and the gorilla appeared in a corner of the room, then moved menacingly toward him. He then sobbed bitterly and talked about his father—"that son of a bitch, he was nice to everybody else and they liked him, but he used to beat us."
>
> At this point his reaction in the psychophysiological laboratory was explained to him as a reactivation of infantile fears and conflicts which had appeared in the form of his old night terrors because of the fatigue and the stress of seven days of sleeplessness. The other subjects, who had observed most of this episode, joined in the discussion that followed and were most understanding and helpful, proving to be most competent cotherapists. After a few minutes he asked that he not be taken from the experiment "because of a little thing like that." He went on to tell that the "Humpty Dumpty-Gorilla" visions had occurred during the previous runs but he had been too ashamed to report them. In the run following this panic episode he again pulled the electrodes off and bolted from the subject room but calmed down quickly after he had left the darkened room. The next run took place without incident and he reported that he had "whipped" his problem. (R. Pasnau et al., "The Psychological Effects of 205 Hours of Sleep Deprivation," *Archives of General Psychiatry*, vol. 18, 1968, pp. 501–502.)

As for the milder disturbances emerging from sleep deprivation, many if not all seem accountable for in terms of very strong sleep tendencies. This results in lapses into borderline sleep, or conflicts which are the consequence of maintaining wakefulness against these strong sleep tendencies. Sleep is a moving away from environmental controls. It is certainly characterized by lowered attention and lowered motivations to do what the environment suggests or demands. With a drift into sleep the person is essentially independent of the environment and may be dominantly responding to an internal transient stimulus. All of us have experienced this as we drift into sleep "dreamlets" or hypnogogic reveries (Chapter 13) that may be quite "real" but not really environmentally there.

When these "drifts" are combined with a totally unreal set of bodily feelings resulting from fatigue, rhythm changes, and a strange laboratory demand that the subject not sleep when every biological force is in the direction of sleep, the surprise lies in the relatively small number of unreal responses occurring. It is even more remarkable that these "oddities" of behavior seldom appear before three days of deprivation and are seldom the most dominant behaviors even after five or six days without sleep.

Performance changes are even less apparent. By "performance" we mean the measurement of performance on a specific task. *The Human Engineering Handbook* developed by the Office of Naval Research was the result of a five-year intensive search of the literature relative to "man-performance" interrelations. Its 1952 edition summarized the effects of sleep loss on performance as follows:

> ". . . there are no effects on the visual and auditory sense functions . . . body steadiness and reaction time are impaired but no other changes in motor control or performance have been noted . . . ability to do mental arithmetic, take an intelligence test, or do memory tasks is affected sometimes, but very frequently scores remain constant . . . complex performances show no clear-cut deterioration . . . subjective attitude is the only factor severely affected. . . .

In short, the effect of sleep loss on performance could hardly be considered devastating.

Careful research since the 1950s has begun to clarify and specify more precise effects. After prefacing his review by saying that factors "have been identified but only a few are well confirmed experimentally," an author concluded in a 1969 article that long, difficult, and complex tasks were more susceptible to sleep loss whereas self-paced, short, well-learned, interesting tasks and those in which knowledge of results were present were most resistant to sleep loss.

Sorting all the data out, the general conclusions about performance seem to be that highly motivated subjects can perform almost any task that requires a short-term effort. On the other hand, sustained periods of performance will typically show deterioration, particularly if they are routine or "dull." Two major exceptions seem to be tasks that require rapid and complex reaction time and short-term memory tasks. These latter involve such things as listening to a series of digits and immediately recalling them. Some complex tasks, particularly those requiring an orderly chain of mental operations (hence short-term memory) may be susceptible.

Again, most of the effects on performance seem accountable for in terms of sleepiness as such. The most powerful "theories" to account for response decrements in long-term tasks invoke the presence of "lapses" into low- or no-performance gaps or "sleepiness." Certainly some of the effects may stem from a lowered willingness to perform due to a preference for sleep.

Selective sleep deprivation

Here we are concerned with the loss of a *kind* of sleep. What are the effects if the substructure of sleep is modified by the elimination of particular stages of sleep?

Research in this area began in 1960 with a particularly dramatic experiment reported by William Dement, a prominent sleep researcher at Stanford University. In this experiment he awakened subjects each time they entered Stage 1-REM sleep. They were permitted to go back to sleep after awakening. By this procedure REM sleep was reduced by some 75 percent. This experiment continued for three to seven nights. Later the subjects were awakened an equal number of times from non-REM sleep periods and the results were compared. There were two striking evidences of "REM pressure." The number of awakenings each night to prevent REM sleep sharply increased and on the "recovery night," a night of uninterrupted sleep, the amount of REM sleep significantly exceeded the amounts present before deprivation. In addition, the study reported psychological disturbances such as anxieties, irritability, and difficulty in concentrating "and five subjects developed a marked increase in appetite."

This study spawned a multitude of offspring. By 1971 there had been at least 40 studies of humans and 40 studies of animals involving literally hundreds of humans and hordes of animals. Most of the studies confirmed the presence of "REM pressure"—the insistence by REM sleep of its place in sleep as evidenced by increased difficulties in suppressing it and a "rebound" on recovery. The search for psycholog-

ical disruptions has not met with a similar success. Basically three
questions have been explored again and again. Does REM deprivation result in personality disorganization? Does REM deprivation
enhance certain generalized or specific drives or motives? Does the
lack of REM impair learning or memory?

In a careful review of all the studies available I concluded as
follows:

**"Is REM necessary for the integrity of the personality or
functional responsivity?** There have been no clear-cut cases in which
RD (REM Deprivation) has resulted in a markedly disorganized
personality response either in normal or in psychotic subjects, who
may be thought to be particularly susceptible to personality disorganization. Similarly, after prolonged deprivation animals have failed to
provide evidence of disrupted functioning. Where some signs of
disorganization have been noted, these findings have been fraught
almost inevitably with the dangers of subject or experimenter
expectancies and/or stressful experimental conditions.

**Does REM deprivation result in a higher need for "drive"
discharge?** Again, in human subjects there have been some subtle
signs of variations in motivational states. However, these have not
been found on objective testings and the most carefully controlled
findings have been essentially negative. Animals have shown some
evidence of increased hunger, sexual drive, and aggression. However,
the responses are similar to those noted in more generalized stress
paradigms and, procedurally, stress is a necessary corollary of RD
animal experiments. In almost all positive instances the "seek and ye
shall find" potential was high.

Is REM sleep critical in learning and memory processing? In the
area of verbal learning, both in regard to learning of new material and
retention of material learned prior to RD, the weight of evidence is to
the contrary. The animal studies are severely compounded by
methodological problems and the data is highly conflictual.

In overall summary, in reviewing all the evidence, I would feel that
a jury would bring in a verdict of "not guilty." There would be worries
about a considerable amount of "circumstantial evidence."

I, of course, may be wrong. Studies continue at a somewhat slowed
pace and the purported effects have become more subtle and complex.
However, a few items about REM that we have met in passing tend to
support my more benign view of REM deprivation. Few of the
purported effects are seen with the total loss of REM under conditions
of total sleep deprivation (above). REM variations are in no apparent
way related to wide variations in psychic changes; schizophrenics and
mental retardates show little or no differences from normals, the vast

changes of personality and learning from the teens to the seventies occur under a very steady REM rate. On the other hand, people with relatively high REM amounts show no discernible differences from individuals with low REM amounts. Within the animal kingdom, REM proportion occupies widely different bands that seem unrelated to intelligence, learning, drives or organization of behavior; the opossum has somewhat more REM than man and the cat somewhat less, for example.[1]

But what of the effect of drugs? Much was made of the disruptive effect of drugs on sleep due to their suppression of the REM stage. These results, as I view them, are effects *on the sleep process itself* and a careful rereading will show no claim for REM suppression on the waking state as such. The strong REM pressure resulting from REM suppression has been consistently reaffirmed. A person taking a suppressor drug, as noted previously, is creating a perpetual battlefield nightly between REM attempting to maintain its integrity and the drug exerting its suppression effect. Broken sleep is a reasonable consequence but a carryover into waking life does not necessarily follow.

A few studies have been performed on Stage 4 deprivation. In these studies there has been a similar stage-specific pressure. Stage 4 is more and more difficult to keep out as deprivation continues—even more so than REM sleep. There is also a "rebound" effect during recovery sleep although this is less sharp than REM sleep and recovery to baseline sleep levels of Stage 4 is more rapid. These few studies have failed to establish any specific behavioral consequences of deprivation periods of up to seven days.

Again, previously noted findings are suggestive in supporting a lack of remarkable effects from an absence of Stage 4. We noted that nearly one-third of 50-year-olds may have *no* Stage 4 sleep (Chapter 4). We would add here that we have not been able to establish a difference in functioning and behavior between those with and those without Stage 4.

Partial sleep deprivation

Of all the forms of sleep deprivation we undergo, the partial loss of sleep is by far the most common. There is almost no one who has not

---

[1] It is of passing interest to note the powerful effect of a single dramatic and logically acceptable study. In question periods after talks or in casual discussion of sleep an almost certain item of "knowledge" about sleep is that "the loss of dream sleep will be very upsetting." Some ten years of generally negative results have a very long way to go in "catching up" with and changing this idea.

at some time been forced by circumstances or made the choice to sharply reduce his amount of sleep. More often than not, this is for one night or perhaps two. Some individuals, however, again by necessity or choice, go on "short rations" for longer periods of time. In addition, there are the many insomniacs, previously discussed, who cannot get as much sleep as they wish.

This discussion of the most common form of deprivation follows the more unusual forms—total deprivation and selective deprivation—for two reasons. First, it combines the two forms of deprivation. It is on the one hand an absence of sleep such as occurs in total deprivation, but on the other it is also a selective deprivation. You may recall the facts noted in Chapter 3 that the substructures of sleep are not uniformly distributed across a normal sleep period and that partial deprivation results in a differential deprivation of REM sleep (Chapter 5). This is because deep sleep (Stage 4) occurs predominantly in the first third of the night and REM sleep occurs with increased amounts in the last third.

A second reason for delaying our consideration of this form of deprivation has been so that we could seek out the effects of the more extreme conditions before we turned to the less extreme. If large and particular effects occur under the extreme conditions, we can look for them more specifically under the less extreme conditions. If the effects of extreme conditions are mild or absent, then effects from the less extreme conditions are not likely to be greater.

Because reduced sleep is so common it is surprising to find such a limited collection of data on the problem. Prior to the 1960s there were 6 studies using reduced sleep regimes. These ranged from one-day-shortened regimes to one week, and the largest used 5 subjects. The total number of subjects studied from the beginning study in 1916 was 15. The reported results, of course, are meager and mixed. They ranged from actual improvement in performance after sleep reduction to subjectively reported low performance. One study in particular exemplified a problem common to them all. In this study subjects were awakened after two, four, six, or eight hours and tested. A decremental effect of short sleep on "body steadiness" and ability to check off two numbers out of a series of numbers was found. It is impossible, however, to know in this instance whether the results stemmed from the shortened sleep period or the "circadian" effect on performance, that is, the general reduction on efficiency resulting from performing the tasks during the usual sleep period.

In the last decade there have been seven studies on this problem and because the question is a central one they should be considered in some detail. Four of these studies concentrated on the effects of shortened sleep on sleep itself. They involved "shortened" sleep regimes of from four to seven days. The results are in complete agreement. Up to a reduction of two hours of normal sleep (about five hours of sleep being permitted) there is no loss of deep sleep (Stage 4) but a significant reduction in REM sleep. With reduction down to four hours of sleep or less there is an actual increase in deep sleep and an even greater, disproportionate effect on REM sleep. On recovery there is the REM "rebound" effect and a curious rebound of Stage 4, or deep sleep, although there has been little or no loss of deep sleep. In longer restricted regimes there are signs of REM sleep "moving forward" in the sleep period; under the pressure of deprivation it begins occurring earlier in the night.

There was evidence of performance effects. In a study of three hours of sleep per night using short term tasks, our laboratory found "evidence of a performance decrement after the seventh and eighth night" of the sharply restricted regime. The decrements were, however, "neither uniform nor fully consistent." But using a "vigilance task" (the monitoring of an infrequent change in tone for a half hour) which has been found to be most sensitive to total sleep deprivation, a researcher found that a single night of three hours of sleep did not have a significant effect but that two successive nights had a clearly significant effect. Indeed, two nights in which sleep was reduced by two hours (five-hour sleep periods) gave some evidence of an effect on a prolonged vigilance task.

Of particular relevance is a study concerned with a "chronically" restricted regime. Our laboratory placed 16 young men on a five-and-a-half-hour sleep schedule for eight weeks. They were typically seven-to-eight-hour sleepers. Once a week they slept in the laboratory and were given an elaborate battery of tests. Each day they completed a questionnaire.

Of the 16 subjects, 15 completed the study. One subject disqualified himself because he required a daily nap to continue the regime. The sleep data was as expected. There was a slight increase in deep sleep and, although there was a tendency to increase the amount of REM sleep in the five-and-a-half-hour period, the REM deprivation was nearly 25 percent of baseline. A number of performance and personality measures showed no effect. A sensitive "vigilance" task showed a significant decline but internal analysis indicated that this was not a decline in "capacity" but in "motivation." Behaviorally, the self-reports showed a significant increase in difficulty getting up in the mornings. Early in the experiment daytime drowsiness was reported, but by the eighth week this was not different from baseline ratings. None reported difficulties in staying up until the appointed time for sleep. We concluded as follows:

> Our study, of course, does not speak to more sharply restricted regimes or more chronic ones. However, the study does suggest that less extreme regimes in terms of either sleep restriction or chronicity are unlikely to result in performance decrements or personality disturbances. These findings further imply that a few hours of transient or even chronic sleep loss of a relatively extended period resulting from work requirements, personality disorders, or insomnias are not likely *per se* to result in major behavioral consequences. The individual's personal reactions to these sleep losses, however, are another matter. At least our findings indicate that he may be reassured about the sleep loss itself.

Implications

We are in the midst of a major puzzle and a great disappointment for the sleep researcher. The puzzle is this: we all *know* that if we can't sleep we're not as well off as we would like to be. However, when we put the problem under the close scrutiny of the laboratory studies of either total, partial, or selective deprivation the effects are far from impressive. The disappointment is obvious. We (the sleep researchers) would very much like to establish that the effects of sleep variations on performance are great and devastating. Unfortunately, this is difficult to prove and difficult to account for relative to what we all know.

A brief review of the experimental facts gives us this picture. Very prolonged sleep loss—five to ten days, for example—yields physiologically only "modest and subtle" effects. The only apparent ones are a hand tremor, occasional double vision, droopy eyelids, a lower pain threshold, and a change in the alpha rhythm; the latter may be simply a sign of intrusive tendencies to sleep. In terms of performance, under prolonged absence of sleep short-term tasks, particularly sensory, motoric, or well-organized ones, seem essentially unimpaired. Complex reaction time, short-term memory, and the ability to sustain low-demand or uninteresting performances show some effect. Behaviorally, while there are occasional and transient evidences of confusion, disorientation, and irritability, the personality is generally intact. The dominant factor is an overwhelming need to sleep and an associated struggle with this need. All of these "disturbances" are sharply limited with one or two nights of loss of total sleep.

How can we account, first, for the relatively limited effects? A most probable explanation is that we are built with a strong "reserve" to the extent that our basic functioning is unimpaired by sleep loss. Let us use an analogy that we are even more familiar with. Suppose we keep a person from eating for, say, three days. What do you expect would happen to his general physiology—heart rate, blood pressure, and the like? His brain and central nervous system? His memory or his motor and sensory controls? I would suggest: very little. Research bears this out. He would, of course, be very hungry and there would probably be some predictable behavior changes. He might well "feel" bad. He might be irritable (How did I get myself into this mess?) or frightened (Am I hurting myself? Will I ever get food again?). He probably would be obsessed by food and even "misperceive" or "hallucinate" about food. But would he show a disturbed or disorganized or psychotic personality? Could you measure basic performance and personality changes? I doubt it.

The sleep experiment is complicated by the fact that sleep is always a constant possibility and persistently there. A starvation experiment, to be equivalent, would require the constant and tempting presence of food. However, I think the analogy makes its point. We can well survive five or more days without food. Why not sleep loss?

But how are we to account for the discrepancies between the experimental findings and our own certain knowledge that to function well we must not go without sleep? First we would note that there are real effects of going without sleep. Although the fundamental functions of the organism do not seem markedly affected, feelings and moods are affected and task persistence is less. Furthermore, there is one certain effect—the person is very sleepy. In fact, this latter certainly may account for most of the poor feelings and performance changes.

The need to sleep and the act of sleeping reflect the need and the deed of not continuing one's effective engagement in the waking world. If there is a very strong need to sleep and this is opposed by a need to stay awake, the result is conflict. The consequences of conflict can take many forms: irritability and aggressiveness, anxiety, or a variety of compromises—rationalizations ("Who *could* do well feeling as sleepy as this?") or conversions ("I could do it if I didn't feel sick at my stomach."), among others.

If the need to stay awake is not strong, the most likely response is sleep: "I'll just take a quick nap and feel better." If the need to stay awake is strong but the need to sleep even stronger, the struggle may be lost fully or intermittently to lapses into sleep. In the latter instances these may be brief and confusing—"Where am I?" or "What was I doing?"

To this effect of real sleepiness we would add several other potential contributors to our "feeling" or "doing" badly under sleep loss. First, a very common observation in sleep-loss experiments is that the worst "behavior" is present during the late-night or early-morning hours. Again and again subjects report things going "okay" during the day of regular activities but "troubles" beginning around 3:00 A.M. or so. They are exhibiting the biorhythm aspect of sleep and waking—the fact that there is a time to sleep and a time to wake (Chapter 5). With or without deprivation we have sharper sleep tendencies and poorer performance during the normal sleep time. Our lessened ability to study or stay awake at 3:00 A.M. is there even if we didn't get up until noon and we have been awake for only 15 hours. Part of our "misbehavior" is simply due to an increase in these natural periods of sleepiness and relative ineffectiveness, not sleep loss.

Whenever we undergo sleep loss we are doing something other than sleeping. In "real life" this is typically in response to a "high-demand" situation. We do not sleep because we cannot or do not want to sleep. This may be some stressful demand—we may be required to complete a report or we may be under some other strong pressure. In these instances our nonsleep is filled with stress and heavy energy output. There may be some positive pursuit of love or amusement. Stress may or may not be present, but energy output is typical and this may well be fueled by a great deal of drinking and smoking.

We are suggesting that often the events taking the place of sleep may account for a reduced efficiency in the system. This is compounded by a "letdown" after the "full push" is over and we are now just trying to "get through the day." Sleep loss may be a very junior partner as a "cause" of our poor feelings in such circumstances.

Finally, there is the matter of expectancies. Nearly everyone believes that sleep loss is bad. This only varies in degree; some believe that the loss of sleep has a very significant effect on how they function and others believe this to a lesser degree. These beliefs roll out the red carpet for any slight feeling of discomfort or signs of inefficiency to walk along: "I'm not doing well—I would have if I'd gotten enough sleep." Certainly some of the discrepancy between our laboratory studies and real life derives from this factor. In the laboratory we "expect" our subjects to do well and they do; in "real life" we do not expect to do well and we do not.

If, then, extreme loss of sleep has a limited effect, can partial sleep loss or loss of particular sleep stages be far ahead in their effects on performance? Logic and data certainly suggest otherwise.

Nearly 100 studies involving the experimental deprivation of sleep stages have primarily resulted in a retreat from the original presumption of remarkable effects to more and more subtle assumptions about the effects of deprivation. There is only very limited evidence that either REM deprivation or slow-wave sleep deprivation results in personality disorganization, motivational changes, or problems in cognitive or motoric functioning. While REM "pressure" or a slow-wave "pressure" has been established, its primary effect seems to be on sleep itself rather than on waking performance.

The experimental studies of partial sleep loss, which we have seen is also a differential deprivation of REM sleep, are considerably less in number. At the same time we can be sure that the "nonexperimental" or real-life "experiments" with partial sleep loss are manifold. Either voluntarily or involuntarily (for example, in the insomniac) individuals shorten their sleep for varying periods of time. The experimental results are clear. A limited reduction of sleep—from seven and a half to five and a half hours for eight weeks—had two effects: the subjects had a hard time getting up in the mornings and showed a lowered capacity to continue to monitor a repetitive signal over a half-hour sequence. Other tests showed no effect.

Many of us know from our own personal experience and our observations of others that there are times when we don't get "enough sleep." Are we worse off for this? We have to guess here, of course, and my guess is no. I say this for two reasons. First, very marked sleep losses show few damaging effects, and they seem worse than they are (above). Second, sleep has a power of its own. It struggles to assert its rights. If we are being significantly affected by a limited curtailment of sleep, it is very possible that we simply will be forced to get a survivable amount somehow.

But does all this mean that we don't have to worry about getting sleep? If sleep loss or disturbance doesn't seem to do bodily harm, is sleep then just a sort of a bad habit that we can ignore? The answer is, of course, no. Sleep cannot be ignored or lost without worry or care.

Sleep is a fundamental, built-in way of behaving. It is not something we can choose to do or choose not to do. The research we have reviewed indicates that little or no fundamental "damage" results from the loss of sleep. However, there are three facts that are certain under these circumstances: we will be doing something else instead of sleeping, we will be less capable of responding during the time when we are usually sleeping, and we will be increasingly sleepy. A person who is sleepy is simply not at his best, and the sleepier he is the less effective are his relations to the world around him. We may struggle valiantly against this strong force but ultimately all performance will bend before it.

We have been primarily talking about acute schedules: losses of sleep for several days, losses of REM sleep for a week, losses of some sleep for eight weeks. We seem to be adaptive enough to survive these effects. More chronic regimes may well exceed this "buffering" and take substantial tolls. The data is suggestive; total losses of sleep when extended into a week or more begin to show exaggerated effects, and chronic struggles between drugs and REM sleep ultimately shatter the sleep response itself. Partial losses of sleep across years may well exact a toll, as yet unspecified. We strongly believe that the effects of sleep distortions as they relate to functioning will be found in chronic regimes. Simply, no inherent system with its natural demand charac- teristics can sustain chronic abuse indefinitely. Such systems struggle to cope with impositions upon their limits. Always this is at some cost. If the pressure is maintained long enough, the system fails or the costs to other systems is excessive and the consequences are felt. We do not yet know the ultimate costs of chronic abuse of sleep, but we can certainly believe that they are there.

13

Sleep and dreams

We have so far almost completely ignored that ever-fascinating world of dreams—although in the second chapter we noted in passing that REM sleep and dreams were associated, and we mentioned the presence of nightmares in our chapter on anomalies and drugs. This omission has been intentional since this book is about sleep and, in our opinion, dreams play a limited role in this process. They may occasionally interrupt sleep, they definitely occur during sleep, and their recall after sleep is certainly interesting and perhaps worthwhile. However, as primary determinants of sleep or as functionaries within sleep, their role is less certain. Rudely put, from the point of view of sleep itself dreams may be viewed as merely the foam on the beer.

However, this position is certainly not universally held and dreams have been widely studied within the matrix of sleep research. Further, the position held does not suggest at all that dreams are not meaningful or clinically useful. For these reasons, and because of the subject's intrinsic interest, this chapter is about dream content.

The nature of dreams

Before we begin a discussion of dreams it would be wise for us to know, with a little more certainty than most of us have, just what a dream is like. Since most of us have had dreams of our own this may seem a little strange, but think about it. Although we know our own dreams we certainly cannot directly experience someone else's. All we directly know about dreams is the nature of our own. But are these like the dreams of others? Frequently I am asked a question like, "Do people dream in color?" I often reply by saying, "Do you?" This is usually most unsatisfactory. The questioner, more often than not, looks puzzled or annoyed and may well say, "I was asking about dreams, not me."

What we know about dreams in general, then, is what other people tell us about their dreams. If we happen to be psychoanalysts we have heard a large number of dreams. Most of us, however, know about others' dreams from casual reports ("Hey, I had this funny dream last night") or highly selective ones ("Man, I had this dream I can't forget"). Our other primary sources are visualizations or descriptions of dreams which make some particular point about clairvoyance, psychodynamics, or enhance some movie, poem, or story theme. In short, we know very little about those night-to-night occurrences that make up the full dream world.

The first problem in knowing the dreams of others is that we can never actually see them and must accept a description of them. This bridge between the dream and our knowing is made of words, and words are often hard to come by. The following is an actual transcript of a laboratory dream report.

s: Yes. Yes, I can hear you. Go ahead.

e: Was anything going through your mind?

s: No, I really just, uh, I was dreaming about . . . let me see, a group of college boys walking down the lane, in the lane, in the uh, in the park, singing, and they were outside there in the distance, and there was a group of girls and all, dressed in white sitting on the park benches, uh . . . carrying flowers, I think. Um, it was dark and they were covering, uh, they were wearing white gloves, I remember long, you know, long white gloves . . . and there was, uh, let's see . . . I'm trying to think of the details . . . lots of flowers in the park. Yellow ones, I think. Regular flowers.

e: Did you recognize anybody in the dream?

s: Uh, no. There's nobody I could recognize.

e: Were you in the dream?

s: No, I wasn't. I couldn't particularly single out anybody that I could recognize in the dream. . . . I had to make a special effort to retain the . . . you know, it disappears after a very few seconds, if I don't make a constant effort to retain it.

e: Were there any feelings connected with it?

s: No. I, uh, I guess you might say I was a passive observer of the scene. I had no feelings either way of what was going on. It had been going on maybe a few minutes, I guess, then I woke up. At the beginning, sometime earlier, it had something to do about insects, uh, bees. I was catching bees. Somebody was catching bees and letting them go on flowers, you know, pollinating the flowers, and uh . . . and uh, uh, I don't know. Could you ask me another question?

E: Did you say you were catching the bees?

S: At first, in the beginning, they were . . . uh, they were in a laboratory or something being used to . . . for experimental purposes. They were being used to pollinate flowers, well that was way back, hard to remember the beginning of the dream. As you go along you get more involved, um, one thing leads to another. Yes, that's about it, you know. These bees were pollinating these flowers, and uh . . . they were bright yellow, shining almost in the dark, and uh, these girls didn't want to see, uh, these boys to see them. They didn't want to see them, so they were trying to hi—to cover up their elbows and holding their arms so that they wouldn't be seen, the gloves wouldn't be seen. The whiteness of the gloves wouldn't be seen in the dark. . . . Way off in the distance you could hear them singing as they were walking along the walks. . . . That's about it.

E: You said it was dark?

S: Yes, very dark.

E: Do you remember what you were dreaming just when you woke up?

S: Yes. At that point they were walking in the distance singing with, uh, the girls sitting on the benches in the foreground listening, and clutching their elbows . . . trying to keep, I think the bright flowers from being seen, you know. Sort of, I think there was possibly a glow, a yellowish glow on the flowers where the bees had been around previously. . . . I guess that's it. (H. Witkins and H. Lewis, "Presleep Experience and Dreams," in *Experimental Studies of Dreaming*, eds. H. Witkins and H. Lewis [New York: Random House, 1967], pp. 164–65.)

Here is a second one from a young librarian:

"I was in the library and I was filing cards, and I came to some letter between 'a' and 'c.' I was filing some, I think it was Burma, some country, and just as I put that in, there was some scene of some woman who was sent to look for a little girl who was lost, and she was sent to Burma. They thought the little girl was going there for some reason. This was sort of like a dramatization of what I was doing. I mean I was filing, and then this scene took place, right at the same time. In the setting it was sort of like you'd imagined it, but I had a feeling that it was really happening. (David Foulkes, "Theories of Dream Formation and Recent Studies of Dream Consciousness," *Psychological Bulletin*, vol. 62, 1964, 244–45.)

There are many aspects of these "raw materials" of dreams. I will point up a few of them. They are very different in clarity and coherence of recall. We can guess that the first dream may not have even been retained as a dream "in real life"; at best, there might have been a vague recall of having had a dream about "being in a park." Second, note the shifting participant roles. In the first dream there was a shift from being an observer to an earlier active role of catching bees, and from passively observing to "knowing" that the girls were hiding their elbows. In the second dream there was a dramatic shift from filing cards to "some woman" to "they" who "thought." Most particularly, note that though strange in many ways, the dreams were populated with real and imaginable events and people: college boys, white gloves, bees, flowers, file cards, Burma, a little girl. While much of the dreams were "as if," they were also composed of "as."

Remember that these dream reports were very close to their sources. A second problem of knowing dreams lies in the recall of the recall. What we finally hear of a dream is very likely to be different from the original dream. Again and again studies have shown that reports of "home dreams" occurring outside the laboratory are very different from those reported in the laboratory. The "home" dreams are more coherent, sexier, and generally more interesting than those reported in the laboratory. Certainly some of this may be due to a difference in the dreams themselves. Laboratory dreams are essentially "random" samples while home dreams are usually final-awakening dreams. Much of the difference is likely to stem from the recall process itself. Freud used the term "secondary elaboration" to describe the pressures toward rationality and the repression which works to modify the original recall. Then, there is simply the matter of what we remember and whether we try to remember. In our examples we may well have received no report at all from the first dream and our second dream would have probably been something like "I dreamed about a little girl who was lost" or "I dreamed about a little girl who was kidnapped and taken to Burma."

Given these limitations, what are the dreams of "people" like? Fortunately, we have two reports which have extensively described and categorized dream content "noninterpretively." One set was composed of 1,000 "home" dreams of college students collected from dream logs by Dr. Calvin Hall,[1] and one set was composed of 650 laboratory dreams collected by Dr. Fred Snyder.[2] In describing

[1] Calvin S. Hall and R. L. Van de Castle, *The Content Analysis of Dreams* (New York: Appleton-Century-Crofts, 1966).

[2] Fred Snyder, "The Phenomenology of Dreaming," in *The Psychodynamic Implications of the Physiological Studies on Dreams*, eds. Leo Madow and Laurence H. Snow (Springfield, Ill. and Charles C Thomas, 1970).

dreams I have drawn heavily from the latter study, since its results are likely to be closer to the "raw" dream itself; I have used the Hall study to elaborate, confirm, and occasionally disagree with the laboratory reports.

The most striking conclusion of both studies is that dreams do not conform to the common assumption that they are generally bizarre, highly unusual, and emotion-laden. Snyder says "Our data . . . entirely conforms to this [Hall's] conclusion that the outstanding feature of dream settings is their commonplaceness." Snyder reports that in only 20 percent of the dreams was the setting not clear, and three-fourths of these dreams were very short reports. In only 4 percent of the dreams was the setting exotic or unusual and less than 1 percent of the settings were classifiable as "fantastic." In the remaining dreams the scenes were familiar, identifiable, or most reasonable.

Dreams are not lonely. In 95 percent of the dreams analyzed by Hall another person beside the dreamer was present, and in 35 percent more than one other person was present. More than half the people were recognizable and familiar to the dreamer. Animals appeared occasionally but only one "monster" appeared in the 1,000 dreams. Notables such as movie stars, sports figures, or politicians were quite rare.

There is a great deal of activity, but this activity is surprisingly unstrenuous. Some 38 percent of the activity involves talking, listening, looking, or thinking. Another 32 percent consists of going from one place to another—walking or riding (but seldom floating). Only about one-fourth of the dreams were about physical activities, and these were mostly recreational. Here dreams do indeed differ from real life in that we seldom find the dreamer working at routine daily tasks of typing or cleaning or repairing or doing manual labor.

Dreams often have dramatic themes. We can categorize these along various dimensions. Dreams of misfortune and failure are more frequent than ones dealing with good fortune and success; their respective percentages were 46 and 17 percent in the Hall sample. There was evidence of aggression in 47 percent of the dreams and friendly encounters in 38 percent. As a special form of friendliness (or aggression) overt sexual behavior was quite rare. In the Snyder study only 6 of the 620 dreams contained overt sexual acts; in the 1,000 dreams analyzed by Hall only 76 displayed sexual behavior and these included sexual fantasies, overtures, kissing, and "petting." There were only 25 incidences of sexual intercourse.

Emotionality within dreams is remarkably bland even in the face of occasionally highly dramatic events. Snyder writes about his experience with this dimension of dreams.

> I am particularly unsatisfied with our ability to assess the emotional dimension of our dream descriptions. It did not seem difficult at first, for unwittingly we were frequently inferring what would have been the appropriate emotion under the circumstances described. Then we began to encounter reports in which the subject emphatically disavowed any such feelings. For instance, a waiter in a restaurant was making erotic advances to the dreamer's sister, resulting in a fist fight; but he specifically denied any accompanying feelings of anger. The fight just seemed like a necessary social amenity. After a few such instances we started all over again, tabulating emotions only when they were definitely identified by the reporter, and none were identified in more than two-thirds of the narratives.

Of the emotions identified in dreams, unpleasant ones were most prominent. Fear and anxiety were associated with more than one-third of the dream emotions, followed closely by anger.

These reports accord well with my own observation of dreams. On the whole the reports are relatable to the real world. To use Snyder's analogy drawn from art, they are "representational" rather than "surrealistic," with occasional forays into "impressionism." They are populated by real people in real settings performing and acting in patterns of recognizable behavior.

Where, then, does the impression of strangeness, which is certainly a characteristic of dreaming, come from? I would say from three primary sources: 1) A loosened temporal and spatial world, 2) Loosened attentional controls and 3) Less critical evaluations.

The dream world has many aspects of fantasy or imagination. In the dream all things are possible in a physical sense. Time and matter are not bound by their physical properties. Time does not flow inexorably forward and matter is not bound by gravity. The past and the future may have reality in the present, the dead may live, and I can ice skate in Burma. Scenes in dreams may change with remarkable rapidity or awesome slowness. I may be in a park in one instance and a laboratory in the next or, indeed, I can be in parts of both at the same time.

The way I attend to the world when I am awake is selective and purposeful. In reality as I walk through the park I may be attending to my destination, or to the potential of being mugged, or to a pretty girl. I am unlikely to attend to yellow gloves or hidden elbows. If I am filing cards I attend to them and not to a woman in Burma. In my dreams I may attend to minute details, or thoughts in a fashion that seems little dominated by particular purposes or the demands of the surround.

Above all, I am not critical in my dreams. I do not say, "That is not possible" or "Don't believe this" or "How puzzling." Rather, I accept what is there even though the event is physically impossible or even disgusting or frightening.

In summary, dreams do have their strange qualities. However, when their components are placed under the microscope of objective analysis, the particular elements of the dream turn out to be remarkably prosaic.

Viewpoints about dreams

Dreams have evoked a wide range of responses throughout time. This is not surprising in view of the qualities that we noted above. To these must be added several other factors that have lent an air of extravaganza to the dream world.

Mary Calkins, a pioneering scientist, wrote in 1893: "Dreams from which conclusions have been drawn in almost all cases are particularly striking and unusual dreams. . . ." And what a vast reservoir there is from which to draw such striking and unusual dreams. Snyder points out that from the conservative assumptions of three REM periods per night and two dream stories within each period there is a resultant 150,000 dreams *per person* over a life span of 70 years. Or we may note that about one person in three recalls having had a dream the night before. In the United States alone, then, there are over 50,000,000 dreams recalled each waking day! In this light it is somewhat surprising that striking, significant, and unusual dreams fail to deluge us with their mysteries each day.

In addition to the sheer presence of dreams, and hence the high probability of unusual ones, there is a natural tendency to ascribe meaning to the unusual and very strong tendencies of "true believers" or exploiters of human nature to use mysterious things toward their own ends . . . be these stars, eclipses, unidentified flying objects, death, or dreams.

The many viewpoints that have emerged across time and cultures and within time and cultures can be grouped generally into four variations: Dreams are seen as a different reality or life; as omens or determinants of waking life; as reflections of waking life; as functional biological systems. Although these general classifications will miss a few of the more exotic attitudes, and they are often not fully discrete in a particular dream stance, they can portray the bulk of the panorama of dream attitudes.

Dreams as another reality: This belief manifests itself in viewpoints ranging from the acceptance of dreams as a different plane of reality, through dreams being thought of as a co-reality with waking life, to tangled philosophical theories in which dreams play a major role.

In many primitive groups, for example the Eskimos of Hudson Bay and the Pantani Malay people, it is thought that one leaves one's body during a sleep period and enters another world. The Tajal people of Luzon established severe punishments for awakening a sleeper lest the "soul" become lost from the body. In many tribes and peoples the dream world has a co-reality with waking, and actions taken in the dream are seen to have the same force and meaning as waking actions. Among such widely different cultures as the Kurdish, Kamchatka, Borneo, or Zulu, to dream of adultery is to be an adulterer; an offense received or given in a dream is an offense received or given in waking, and a gift given or taken in a dream requires recompense in waking.

Philosophers have often speculated about the reality base of the dream. In the third century B.C., the Chinese philosopher Chuang Tzu clearly posed the dilemma. He had dreamed that he was a butterfly, ". . . conscious only of my fancies as a butterfly." Suddenly he awoke and posed the problem of whether he was a butterfly dreaming that he was a human or a human dreaming that he was a butterfly. Bertrand Russell put it more bluntly: "I do not believe that I am now dreaming but I cannot prove that I am not."

Dreams as omens: One of the oldest and most persistent beliefs about dreams is that they have a prophetic character. One of the earliest writings in book form is an Egyptian papyrus in the British Museum dating from 1350 B.C. It is about dream interpretations. Today one can buy "dream books" in New York to predict the proper number to play in the numbers lotteries.

Throughout history and literature the prophetic tradition is strong and rife with familiar examples. In the *Odyssey* dreams play a frequent role. Alexander the Great proceeded to take Tyros after having had a dream about a satyr. His dream interpreter ascribed to the dream the meaning "Tyros is thine," from a play on the words *sa Tyros*. The Old Testament details the roles of Joseph and Daniel in interpreting the dreams of the Pharaoh and Nebuchadnezzar after their court interpreters had failed. There are significant references to dreams in the New Testament also. In reference to the birth of Jesus:

> But while he thought on these things, behold the angel of the Lord appeared unto him in a dream, saying, "Joseph, thou son of David, fear

not to take unto thee Mary thy wife; for that which is conceived in her is of the Holy Ghost"

and

"Behold, the angel of the Lord appeareth to Joseph in a dream, saying, Arise, and take the young child and his mother and flee to Egypt. . . ."

Today interest and belief in the prophetic or omen dream is still quite active. There is almost certainly a large assortment of books purporting to teach you how to predict the future from your dreams at your neighborhood newsstands and in bookstores. For a short time I tried collecting them but, having acquired nearly a dozen in three trips out of town, I gave up. I found that they rank closely behind the books on astrological predictions.

Beyond these books, dreams which project the future are at the center of many parapsychological issues. In the early works of the Society for Psychical Research, before the influence of the experimental approach toward ESP, clairvoyant and predictive dreams were, in fact, the most prominent focuses of such studies.

Of course, the clarity and accuracy of prophetic dreams vary widely. The *Odyssey* speaks of false dreams, which pass through "the gates of Ivory" and true dreams, which pass through "the gates of Horn." The ancient and religious literature contains many "message" dreams which were attributable to a god or heroic figure. As reported, the message was typically clear and unequivocal. There are many clear predictive dreams described post hoc in the psychic literature. However, most predictive dreams require interpretation and in cultures where predictive dreams are valued, interpreters, often priests or elders, are almost inevitable and powerful.

Dreams as reflections of waking life: From this perspective, dreams are not considered to be a form of reality or predictive but are considered to be reflections of the life of the dreamer. This is essentially a naturalistic position, holding that the dream is essentially an "echo" of a point in the individual's waking world which is "heard" in the dream world. The particular position varies generally along two dimensions: the nature of the antecedent event or events and the amount of active "dream work" on this particular source.

The great early Greek philosopher Aristotle presented in some detail a "reflective" theory of dreaming. He stated that we perceive events in our sleep just as we perceive events while awake. While we are awake, perceptions result from the stimulation of our senses. However, when we are awake, impressions of sensory events can continue and be perceived after the original event has passed. So, too, can these impressions persist into sleep. Whether from external or internal sources of stimulation, they may occur with even "greater impressiveness" in sleep because the "intellect" during sleep is not working together with the senses. Furthermore, the original sensory events, "like eddies in a great river, often remaining as they were when first started [are often] broken into other forms by collisions with other objects." Aristotle also noted the effects of emotions in modifying the received sense impressions. This theory of dreams, which includes considerable speculation about "dream work," is all the more remarkable when we realize that it was put forth in a time when the dominant notions about dreams were that they were oracular or curative, representing visitations from the gods. During this period there were well over 600 dream temples where, after appropriate sacrifices to the gods, people slept and sought interpretations or direct interventions to "cure" their ailments or direct their lives.

The emergence of the scientific attitude accelerated naturalistic or materialistic beliefs about dreams. Thomas Hobbes, an early English philosopher, wrote on dreams in the 1650s. He considered that dreams reflected the presence of imagination in sleep, and that these imaginations (as all imaginations) were the results of earlier sense events. Particular dreams, for Hobbes, evolved from stimulations of various kinds occurring to the sleeper: ". . . as Anger causeth heat in some parts of the Body when we are awake; so when we sleep, the overheating of the same parts causeth Anger, and raise up in the Brain the Imagination of an Enemy." The position that particular dreams were evoked by immediate sensory events reached a climax in the works of the French physician Maury, who studied more than 3,000 dreams in the 1860s. He would experimentally tickle a person with a feather or sound a bell and ask the now-wakened sleeper about his dream. He concluded that dreams were forgotten memories that were unlocked or elicited by external stimuli.

It was Sigmund Freud in his landmark book, *The Interpretation of Dreams*, written in 1900, who brought the reflective theories of dreams to a striking fruition. Freud asserted that all dreams were meaningful and were reflective of important aspects of the individual psychodynamic needs. There were three basic aspects of Freud's interpretive system:

1. The recalled dream was the *manifest content* of the dream, which was derived from events of the day (day residue), physiological states during sleep such as bladder tension, and infantile memories.

2. The manifest content expressed a *latent content* of wish fulfillment

dealing with unfulfilled unconscious sexual wishes. These in turn were primarily the result of unresolved early childhood psychosexual development.

3. The latent content was understandable in terms of "dream work," which transformed the latent content into a manifest content that was "acceptable" to the dreamer.

In this framework the dream was a "guardian" of sleep. Through "dream work" the latent and repressed sexual wishes were modified into an acceptable manifest content which made use of the current aspects of life.

Freud emphasized four basic dream work mechanisms: condensation, displacement, symbolization, and secondary elaboration. The first three of these result from the fact that dreams express themselves through imagery rather than words. Because of this, logical relations such as "either-or," "because," or "although" that are available in speech are not present in dreams. A dream cannot "say": "This scene is related to the following scene because . . ." Rather, one scene simply follows another and their relationship must be discovered. In a dream it is not a matter of "either this or that"; the "either" and the "or" appear without conjunction. Expressions and feelings must be presented pictorially. The dream cannot say "I dislike you"; it must "do something" to show "dislike." It cannot say "I am sad"; it must portray sadness by tears or, perhaps, funerals. The dream work of condensation, displacement, and symbolization involves this use of imagery toward its logical ends.

In condensation a single image may come to represent a highly involved and complex relationship. Freud gives as an example one instance of condensation from a fragment of a short dream by an older woman patient of his. She dreamed that a beetle was crushed as she shut a window on it. She had become much concerned about the waning of sexual relationships with her husband. She had become aware that crushed beetles were thought to be a powerful aphrodisiac. This image was a condensation of these complex thoughts and wishes.

Displacement occurs when an emphasis of the dream is detached and displaced to some other aspect of the dream. This may be an emotional or conceptual displacement. A man may dream of a rebuff by a girl who is particularly unattractive; this may be representative of the failure of an important homosexual liaison. This would be a double displacement of the emotional disappointment and the homosexual relationship.

Symbolism played a significant role in Freud's dream interpretation schema. In symbolism, as in condensation and displacement, abstract terms and concepts are reduced to concrete representations. Since Freud contended that dreams were primarily sexual in origin, concrete objects frequently "stood" for sexual acts or parts: "All elongate objects, such as sticks, tree trunks, umbrellas (the opening of these being comparable to an erection) may stand for the male organ—as well as all long sharp weapons . . . Boxes, cases, chests, cupboards and ovens represent the uterus, and also hollow objects, ships and vessels of all kinds . . . Steps, ladders or staircases, or as the case may be, walking up and down them are representations of the sexual act. . . ."

On awakening, secondary elaborations occur. In recalling dreams there is the pressure of repression on recall and a search for rationality. Through additions and subtractions, the dream is made more acceptable to the dreamer.

Freud considered the interpretation of dreams to be "the royal road to the unconscious." By deciphering the dream, the core problems of the person could be revealed.

Procedurally Freud relied heavily on the person's free associations to the elements of the dream. From these associations, Freud's other information about the patient, an understanding of the dream work, and an analysis of the dynamics behind the latent content, the meaning of the dream was inferred.

A possible Freudian interpretation of the librarian's dream described earlier in this chapter might follow this course. In free associating to the letter "B" she may have replied "boy" and further associated the name "Bernard." The filing may have been symbolic of sexual relations with a former lover named Bernard. The "lost" child may have represented this love through unresolved relationships with her mother, who was represented by the unrecognized woman in the dream. Freud might have traced the dream back to mother conflict, which was affecting current sexual relations.

The intervening 75 years have amended and elaborated these basic contributions of Freud, but their essence has been retained: dreams are a meaningful reflection of a person's psychological concerns and they are interpretable through a recognition that dreams speak in a variant language form and with a greater freedom in logic and emotions.

The major shifts in emphasis have been fourfold. First, there has been a focus on the meaning, in and of itself, of the manifest content. Rather than considering the recalled dream to be a disguised or evasive statement which has been created to permit the expression of an unacceptable wish, the dream is considered as a direct but dream-form statement of the individual's concern. In short, the dream is not saying one thing and meaning another.

Second, the source of the dream is attributable to the here and now of the dreamer rather than reflecting more infantile or remote sources of conflict. If the dream is about someone that he hates now, it is that person the dreamer hates and not his father.

Third, the dream is taken to express a broader range of underlying problems or aspects of the dreamer's concerns. Rather than expressing simply sexual wish fulfillments, the dreams may express the full range of the dreamer's life: problems, hopes, fears, enjoyments, life-style. His dreams may be simple reminders of current pressures, such as putting off studies for an examination, or may reflect more chronic struggles, such as a growing discontent with growing old.

Fourth, the specificity of the symbolic meaning of the elements or aspects of the dream has been sharply reduced. All aspects of the dream are symbolic but the representation is particular to the person in his time and place. For different persons, boarding a train may either represent a flight from a problem, engaging in a new adventure, worry about car repairs or, simply, a concern about making a plane reservation for an upcoming trip.

As a consequence of these changes, the shift of focus in dream interpretation has been from the dissection of the dream by an analyst to yield information about deep-rooted conflicts of a patient, to an effort by the individual dreamer to understand "the letter written to oneself" with a focus on his present ways of living and coping.

In the librarian's dream, the interpretation and expression of the dream may have simply been that she was bored with her job as a librarian and she wished to find a great new adventure. The particular pursuit to Burma may have resulted from a recent spy movie set in the Far East. Or the dream may have been expressing a conflict between her professional restrictions and her desire for freedom, with the unconscious anxiety about this conflict reflected in the symbolic "lost" child.

Dreams as functional states: These conceptualizations of dreams are concerned with the purpose that dreams serve by their presence. Rather than focusing on their functions in terms of prediction or reflection, researchers in this area ask: "Why do we dream?" Most of this questioning is of quite recent origin. It stems certainly from the very surprising finding that dreaming, as identified by the EEG and eye movements, occurs in all of us and for a great deal of time each night. Before this, dreams seemed to happen or not happen in an unpredictable manner—little or not at all for some people, and more in others; intermittently and varying in degree of clarity and strength within each dreamer. To ask what was the function of such ephemera would be something like asking why some people could carry a tune and others could not, or why some people had moles and others did not. However, when it was discovered that everyone underwent a physiological state that was closely linked to dreaming and that this lasted for more than an hour or so during each night, the question of what it was doing there became a more pressing one.

Before we turn to the answers that have been given we must briefly review some of the more prominent facts that the EEG studies have provided us about dreams during sleep.

The relationship between the EEG and dreams was discovered in 1953. While observing the kinds of eye movements that occurred during sleep in conjunction with the EEG, two scientists at the University of Chicago found that after about 90 minutes the eyes would begin to move very rapidly and the EEG would give the appearance of a "waking" brain although sleep continued. This would last for 10 or so minutes, stop, and then be repeated about 90 minutes later. The experimenters immediately guessed that the person was dreaming and, indeed, on awakening from such periods the subject would very frequently report that he had been dreaming; awakenings from other periods of sleep seldom yielded a dream.

From that study literally thousands of nights of REM-Stage 1 sleep and dream relationships have been examined. We have noted a number of facts about REM sleep in earlier chapters. Some of these will be recapitulated here along with other core findings about REM sleep.

Dreams and REM sleep: In the excitement of the discovery that REM sleep and dreams were coordinate, the initial assumptions were that mental activity, in the form of dreams, was continuous during REM and that the remainder of sleep was "silent." The few failures to recall dreams from REM awakenings were seen as unfortunate accidents and the presence of "dreams" outside of REM was thought to be the recall of a dream which had actually occurred during REM. Research quickly found the matter to be considerably more complicated. The percentage of "dreams" from REM awakening was reported to range from 60 to 88 percent; the percentage of non-REM "dreams" ranged from 7 to 64 percent.

The first thing that became clear was that the percentages depended very much on how one defined a dream. If one required the dream to be a clearly present, visual, storylike event, then almost all such "dreams" occurred with REM awakenings. While the use of this definition reduced or almost eliminated the number of non-REM dreams, it also sharply reduced the number of REM dreams. On the other hand, if one accepted the presence of any mental content— "thinking about something" or a brief or vague recall of "something" —the number of REM and non-REM dreams increased, but the non-REM dreams more so. Taking all mental content into account, awakenings from sleep produce a great deal of ongoing cognition. REM dreams produce more of what we tend to think of as dreams—visual, hallucinatory-type events—while non-REM awakenings produce more "thoughtlike" and realistic material. A person awakened from non-REM may say "I was thinking about my exam tomorrow" or, even, "I wasn't really asleep."

Second, it was apparent that REM and non-REM periods were not independent and homogeneous states. The REM period was not a continuous state of eye movements but had times of high activity interspersed with times of quiescence; further, it was found that there may be brief bursts of REMs outside of the REM state. Hence, there could be non-REM-like recalls within the REM period during quiescence and "dreams" might be transiently present outside of REM periods.

It was seen also that the conditions of awakening and the attempts to capture the mental events could affect the amount of recall. Dreams were more likely to be recalled from abrupt awakenings and without any intervening activity except an intensive effort to recall. Non-REM mental content could be completely missed by asking "Tell me about your dream" instead of "What was going through your mind before you woke up?"

We must further qualify the relationship between this state of REM sleep and dreaming. You will recall that nearly half the sleep of the baby is comprised of REM sleep. The best evidence from premature infants indicates that this state of sleep is even higher before birth. Also we have noted that REM sleep is present in lower animals. In all mammals and even in birds we find this episodic burst of activity within sleep. Unfortunately, we can't ask the newborn or the opossum or the chicken about their dreams. Most of us, however, doubt the presence of "real" dreams in rats and bats, cows and chickens, and unborn children.

The presence, amount, and character of REM sleep: First, it is present in significant amounts. In human adults, from about the onset of adolescence to the sixties, it constitutes about 25 percent of a sleep period. In eight hours of sleep this is more than an hour and a half. There is seldom less than 15 percent—about an hour—or more than 30 percent—over 2 hours.

In babies the proportionate amount of REM is higher—about 50 percent of infant sleep. Since they also sleep longer, the absolute amount of REM is high in a 24-hour period. This averages some 4 out of every 24 hours.

There are wide species differences in the proportionate amount of REM within sleep. Some examples are: opossums—29 percent; cats—25 percent; rats—20 percent; mice—15 percent; rabbits—13 percent; birds—1–3 percent.

In all ages and species REM appears in rhythmic bursts. The time between periods varies with age and species. While the interval between REM episodes in humans averages between 90 and 100 minutes, infants have about a 60-minute cycle, cats a 25-minute cycle, and rats and mice about a 10-minute cycle.

There is increasing evidence that this cycling of REM episodes continues during the waking period but is not detected because it is overridden by our day-to-day functioning.

The amount of REM sleep is systematically affected by a number of conditions. In the early years of life REM diminishes to about 25 percent in the early teens and remains stable into the sixties. Of the time variables, prior wakefulness has a limited effect but displacement of sleep from its regular time of occurrence reduces the latency of REM onset and thereby increases the amount in a given time. Reducing the regular length of a sleep period disproportionately reduces the amount of REM obtained because it is more predominant in the later periods of regular sleep periods. REM sleep is relatively unaffected by "normal" variations in the surround, or by the sleeper's personality or behavior. Indeed, even pathological conditions such as schizophrenia or mental retardation have limited effects on the structure of REM. On the other hand, drugs have a quite marked effect.

In short, REM sleep gives the appearance of a unique state within sleep, revealing highly stable biorhythmic aspects. The primary variables affecting it are temporal (hence rhythmic) distortions associated with the sleep event itself, such as variations in time and length of sleep, and changes within the central nervous system due to aging or use of drugs.

The neurophysiology and physiology of REM sleep: REM sleep is dependent upon a very small structure in the brain stem, the bulge below the neocortex, or gray matter, and below the complex midbrain. This bulge at the top of the spinal cord is known as the pons (See Figure 9-1). A lesion in a very limited area within that section of the brain will eliminate REM sleep while sleep and waking behavior continue to alternate.

This small area spontaneously "fires" or is activated in the approximate 90-minute cycle of REM sleep. With its activation, neural impulses ascend to the upper brain and we see the waking pattern in the EEG. At the same time, as can be most clearly seen in lower animals, there is a descending set of impulses that signal a relaxation of the skeletal muscles. To me this is a marvel of biological adaptation. There is a simultaneous arousal of the central nervous system, which typically results in an increase in behavioral activity, and a "deactivation" of the muscles associated with behavioral activity.

In addition to these central nervous system events there are a number of other physiological accompaniments during REM periods. There are, of course, the rapid eye movements from which REM gets its name. The heart rate and respiration become irregular. In lower animals there is a general loss of muscle tonus, but in addition there may be twitching and jerking of the limbs. The onset of REM is generally associated with a penile erection or an increase in vaginal blood flow.

Distinct biochemical changes associated with the REM periods are also becoming increasingly specified.

In brief summary, contemporary research has closely related the presence of the mental state that we know as dreaming to the presence of a uniquely organized biorhythm of the central nervous system. Its presence within sleep encompasses about one-fourth of sleep time, and it is quite stable and systematic in its responses. It has a particular developmental pattern, is ubiquitous in the animal kingdom, is particularly susceptible to temporal displacements of sleep and to drugs, but is relatively impervious to other variables that affect the other sleep stages. These characteristics have resulted in its being called a "third state"—neither sleeping nor waking.

There have been numerous attempts to ascribe a function or functions to these complex phenomena. The strictly biophysiological approaches have tended to focus on certain descriptive aspects of the REM periods. The "stimulation" theories have suggested that the REM state is a central nervous system "activator" which may be necessary for the development of the central nervous system (pointing to the high amounts in infant sleep) or to offset, in a homeostatic fashion, the reduced level of central nervous system functioning during sleep. Pointing up the strong rhythmic character of REM episodes, biorhythmic notions have inferred some kind of necessary "benchmark" or timing-system involvement. The biochemical theories tend toward restorative conceptions in which the unique biochemical changes result in a rebalancing of the central nervous system.

Physiological approaches have attempted to relate the presence and amount of REM to metabolism, temperature regulation, and ocular functioning. A biological theory has suggested a "sentinel" function of REM—a continuous "alerting" or preparation of action of the animal during the reduced vigilance level associated with sleep.

The psychological models have tended to be more imaginative. Psychoanalytical models and computer models have suggested that dreams may serve to "drain off" repressed impulses or "sort" or "dump" emotional or cognitive content. The more cognitive models have ascribed "memory coding" or "consolidation" or "reorganization" to the REM state.

I must confess that I have found none of the purported functions convincing to date. All are faced with the implacable facts reviewed in the earlier chapters. Behavior does not seem markedly affected by massive deprivations of REM sleep. No strong relationships have been found between extant and palpable differences in emotions and intellect and REM sleep. Schizophrenics, mental retardates, and cats have REM sleep characteristics very much like those of normal human beings. High and low amounts of REM in an individual, either on the average or on a particular night, do not seem predictable by any antecedent or predictive of any subsequent behavior.

In sleep research we are all impressed with the awesome presence of this state and its unique properties. We are increasingly certain of its biochemical, neurophysiological, and descriptive characteristics. However, it would be somewhat surprising if we completely understood its ultimate nature and functions after the 20 short years of its known presence.

Implications

The trailing edge of dreams recalled from the world of sleep has evoked a variety of viewpoints across time and cultures. They have been seen as different forms of existence, as prophecies, and as complex reflections of our waking life. The interpretation of dreams as signs or reflectors of our psychological concerns was given a strong impetus by Freud in the early 1900s. Modern dream research has related dreams to the unique physiological state of REM sleep—a biological rhythm which occupies nearly one-fourth of our sleep time.

The questions "Why do we dream?" and "What do dreams mean?" are multilevel in their implications and in the uncertainty of our answers. At one level we can say that we dream because of an increasingly well-known set of neurological and biochemical changes in our brain. However, a more functional answer to the question is by no means certain. At one level, dreams may be considered a "different" existence. The neurophysiological organization of this event and the thought modes during this time are indeed different. However, there are no new, in-this-time-only biochemical, neurological, or physiological states present, and dreams are populated by real people and placed in a knowable world. While the patterning may be different, the elements are familiar. Similarly, we may view dreams as prophetic. The dreamer is dreaming from and within his time. Just as we can "know" what the future will bring and how we will act with some degree of reasonable certainty in our waking state, so, too, the dream can anticipate that future. However, it seems unlikely that this natural physiological state of the brain can somehow reach into the future and create it in the present.

Certainly the years of clinical study of dreams and the often very clear relationship between the dream and the dreamer's waking life have provided convincing evidence that dreams are reflective. However, methods for "decoding" and sorting out the messages with great certainty have not been fully realized. There has been a decreasing dependence on set meanings for specific symbols or dream aspects, the use of free association, and the view that dreams are restricted in their meaning to limited problem areas such as sex.

The amount, the sturdiness, the orderly patterning, and the ubiquity of the REM phase which is so closely associated with human dream recall—these all attest to the fundamental character of this state. The search continues apace for its full meaning.

14

Why we sleep

Somewhat over 300 years ago, the brilliant English author and essayist Samuel Johnson wrote:

> Sleep is a state in which a great part of every life is passed . . . Yet of this change, so frequent, so great, so general, and so necessary, no searcher has yet found either the efficient or final cause; or can tell by what power the mind and body are thus chained down in irresistible stupefaction; or what benefits the animal receives from this alternate suspension of its active powers. . . . And, once in four-and-twenty hours, the gay and the gloomy, the witty and the dull, the clamourous and the silent, the busy and the idle, are all overpowered by the gentle tyrant, and all lie down in the equality of sleep. . . . (*The Idler*, Nov. 25, 1758)

The ensuing 300 years and the recent intensive assaults on this dark kingdom of the "gentle tyrant" have only begun to modify with certainty some aspects of this evocative statement. We are well on our way, in central nervous system and biochemical terms, to knowing "by what power the mind and body are thus chained down. . . ." I hope that this book will have demonstrated some grasp of the rules by which this "gentle tyrant" governs. However, as for the "efficient and final cause . . . or what benefits the animal receives . . . ," there is as yet little certitude.

Ernest Hartmann, in a recent book, has noted:

> In sleep research, as in other areas of scientific inquiry, *why* is often the first question asked and the last question answered, or left unanswered . . . The scientist usually retreats from the question, considering it either unscientific or too large to tackle. Some scientists

feel that their job is to study only mechanisms, or the *how*, and not functions, the *why*. Others, following Sherrington (1906), have a larger view of science: "Physiology pursues analysis of the relations of the body considered as physical and chemical events; but, further, it aims at giving a reasoned account of the acts of an organism in respect of their purpose and use to the organism *qua* organism." (*The Functions of Sleep* [New Haven: Yale University Press, 1974])

I find it desirable, if not necessary, to present in this chapter a theory of "why" we sleep, that is, a hypothesis as to the purpose of sleep. I do so, primarily, because of the heuristic role that theory has always played in relation to data by organizing facts in a more meaningful and understandable way. Without theory the sheer mass of unorganized and unrelated facts tends to completely obscure the process itself. I hope, then, that this essay into theory will not only give us a better understanding of sleep, but will help to summarize and organize the facts that we have already covered.

The problem

What must a theory "explain" about sleep? We already know that it is an almost universal phenomenon in all animals. While there are a few exceptions, as you move across the panorama of animal life sleep is ubiquitously present, with remarkably common core characteristics: a radically reduced activity level; a lower responsiveness to environmental stimulation; a similar pattern in the central nervous system as reflected in the EEG; a repetition of the changes again and again, every 24 hours. Certainly, then, it must be fulfilling some essential function for life and a theory must speak to that function.

But a decent theory must go beyond an explanation of a common function. The differences in sleep behavior across species are dramatically different. Some animals, like the elephant or cow, sleep very little each day; some animals, like the gorilla or opossum, sleep a great deal. Some animals sleep for long periods of time; some in brief bursts. Some animals sleep at night but others sleep during the day. A theory of sleep must "fit" or help to explain these wide differences in the forms of sleep behavior.

Finally, it should help us understand the function and nature of sleep within our own lives. It must fit that function to the remarkably different forms that human sleep takes. We have seen that human sleep differs across the age span from infancy to old age, and within a given age period among individuals and in relation to circumstances. Whatever it does, the theory cannot violate or ignore these facts.

Sleep as an adaptive response

Fortunately, the theory to be proposed about the function of sleep can be stated rather simply:

Sleep developed, in the particular forms and patterns it took in each species, as a behavior that increased the likelihood of that species' survival. The particular survival value associated with sleeping—that of reducing behavioral activity—was to protect the animal (including man) from dangerous or inefficient activities, both his own and others', particularly in relation to foraging or food gathering. Sleep, then, evolved in each species as a form of "nonbehavior" when *not* responding in the environment would increase survival chances.

I will illustrate what I mean by talking about the possible development of human sleep. In a drastically oversimplified manner, assume for these purposes a population of "humanlike" creatures that tried to operate across the 24 hours without modern "conveniences" of guns and lights. Over generations, we could guess that those creatures that continued to function across the dark period would decrease in number due to death via either the saber-tooth tiger, falls into bogs and off cliffs, or exhaustion from futilely using energy with little payoff. In contrast, those that found safe places to *not* respond during dangerous or ineffective times would survive to produce offspring like themselves and ultimately become the dominant species.

But why sleep? Why not sit in the caves, or around the fires, or in trees or compounds throughout the dark and scheme and build for the future? This part of the argument better fits the more primitive forms of activity and sleep in less developed species, but the point holds for our humanoids. Organisms are "built" to respond to the environment. So long as they are awake they will be active and responsive. In lower species—the rat, for example—you can measure sleep and waking as readily with an activity device as with the EEG. When the animal is awake he is active and "moving" in relation to the environment. Only when he is asleep does activity cease. A part of the theory, then, is that sleep is necessary to "hold" the animal's behavior in check. It is the system that permits the necessary periods of "nonbehaving." The hypothetical survivors of our hypothetical situation were those whose central nervous system "permitted" them to "nonrespond" to the environment by means of sleep.

By stating three basic propositions we can make a number of specific predictions about the wide range in patterns of sleep among species. The three propositions are:

   1. To survive, appropriate "not-responding" is required.

   2. One of the major survival pressures is obtaining a food supply. This is both a positive pressure—to obtain food—and a negative pressure—to avoid being a food supply for predators who are higher in the predatory hierarchy.

   3. Sleep is critical in maintaining these periods of nonresponse.

Let me give a few illustrations from animal sleep for which this scheme seems appropriate. As we have often noted, there are 3 dimensions along which the superstructure of sleep can vary: amount per 24 hours, number (length) of the periods, and placement. Most grazing animals such as cows, sheep, and deer sleep very little in total amount (as little as 2 hours per 24), only in brief bursts, and the nocturnal placement is not sharply fixed; that is, they sleep during both the day and the night. This pattern makes "survival" sense. They sleep very little because "nonbehaving" has low survival value. They have no safe sleeping place—most wander on open plains—and because they are not generally ferocious they are low in the predator hierarchy. To sleep a great deal would mean nonsurvival. Similarly, sleep is intermittent—with no safe sleeping place and in wandering herd behavior, long sleep periods are not possible. The nocturnal effect is not strong because, being herbivorous, the food is in supply throughout the 24 hours.

Elephants also sleep about 2 hours per 24. However, they tend to sleep for a longer single period, and at night. Their limited sleep amount, we would say, is not due to their response to predators but simply due to the amount of foraging necessary for them. Simply, they have to stay active to avoid starving to death. However, when they do sleep, because they are high in the predator hierarchy there is no need for intermittency but their sleep can be set in a longer single period and take place during the night because foraging is somewhat less efficient then. The very tiny short-tailed shrew also has very little sleep although it has a relatively safe sleep environment in a burrow. However, it has an extremely high metabolism rate requiring a food intake of at least its body weight per day if it is to stay alive; to sleep simply would be to court starvation.

On the other extreme, there are animals that sleep a great deal.

The gorilla sleeps about 14 hours per 24. One obvious reason is that it can sleep a long time since it has no predators except man. As a variation on an old joke goes: "How long can a gorilla sleep?" "As long as he wants to!" One important addition is that gorillas also inhabit forest areas where food supply is continuous, so they have no requirements for extensive foraging. For very different reasons, ground squirrels also sleep a great deal—some 14 hours per day. We would attribute this to the safe sleeping environment available in the form of extensive burrows that provide security from predators.

Some animals are crepuscular, active in the early evening and early morning hours. A number of species of the bat family illustrate this pattern. They sleep during the day and the midevening in caves, and fly at dusk and dawn. This seems an excellent illustration of keying the activity-sleep rhythm to the food supply of insects on which they live.

A final illustration. Baboons sleep most adaptively. They retire into nests high in trees at sunset and sleep there until dawn. They then forage alertly and diligently during the day. Their adapted safe place and their long single sleep period remind me considerably of human sleep.

Briefly, what we have proposed as a theory of the function of sleep is this. Each animal inherited—and continues to inherit—a particular pattern of nonresponse to the environment which best fits it to survive relative to its unique physiology and the environment of its evolutionary development. A primary force in shaping these patterns was food gathering (and avoidance of other food gatherers). Sleep serves to maintain this behavior pattern by reducing activity and dampening sensory input, thereby also reducing energy output. Sleep, then, can be thought of as an instinctive response which is useful in "keeping us out of harm's way."

Before turning to an alternative position or extending this notion to our own sleep there should be one addition. Why do we wake up? We would use the same postulates and reasoning that we applied to sleep except in reverse: there is a need *to* respond as well as *not* to respond, and we inherit the appropriate system. Again focusing on food gathering as a positive need, awakening is simply a response appropriately fixed to meet that need. Physiological and neurophysiological cues and mechanisms signal a need and timing for the renewal of food-gathering activities keyed to the animal's ecology. Put simply, the system says, "You need more food to keep going. It's out there and as safe as it's going to be. Get going!" Dr. Seuss has a highly imaginative approach to this problem.

A different theory

The theory of sleep just outlined is very different from the theory that usually dominates our thinking. Ask almost anyone why they

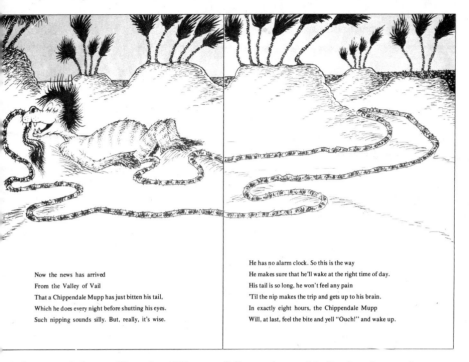

Now the news has arrived
From the Valley of Vail
That a Chippendale Mupp has just bitten his tail,
Which he does every night before shutting his eyes.
Such nipping sounds silly. But, really, it's wise.

He has no alarm clock. So this is the way
He makes sure that he'll wake at the right time of day.
His tail is so long, he won't feel any pain
'Til the nip makes the trip and gets up to his brain.
In exactly eight hours, the Chippendale Mupp
Will, at last, feel the bite and yell "Ouch!" and wake up.

sleep and they will reply: "To rest." Press that a bit further by saying, "That's describing sleep, all right. But why rest?" The answer will usually be: "To recover from our daily labors." This is the "restorative" theory of sleep, which holds that we sleep to recover from the wear and tear of our daily lives; to refurbish our "worn-down" system; to repair our tired bodies. Shakespeare has memorialized this position exquisitely in the phrase "sleep that knits up the ravelled sleeve of care."

This "common-sense" position is supported by considering sleep as "maladaptive," even dangerous. From this it would follow that there *must* be an important restorative function present which occurs in spite of the maladaptive nature of sleep. As put by Walter Hess, one of the great sleep researchers:

> The more differentiated an organism, the more it depends on conscious elaboration of, and appropriate reaction to, signals from the external world in its struggle for survival. During sleep these capacities are depressed and the individual is left defenseless. The fact that all highly organized creatures accept this risk for a considerable part of their life suggests that sleep must have a vital function. We consider it a

reparative process which obviously cannot take place in the higher
centers while they are active. (*Das Zwischenhirn* [Basel, 1954])

Between two theories

The differences between these two theories about sleep may not be
too apparent but they are very real.

The adaptive theory says that we inherit, from an evolutionary
shaping in relationship to the environment, an automatic timing
which determines that we will sleep and awaken in an appropriate
way to the environment. Each 24 hours, rain or shine, busy or idle,
warm or cold, the tendencies to sleep that fit our ecological niche
occur. If we and the world permit it, we will sleep and then awaken to
effectively live in the world again. As an early writer put it, we do not
sleep because we are exhausted but rather to avoid exhaustion.

The restorative theory says that our activities and engagements
each day diminish, destroy, wear out, or drain some energy source and
we sleep in response to this. During sleep there is a restorative process
which prepares us or renews us to engage in the next day's activities.
Although I have never seen it so stated, I think we can assume that
this system is an inherited one and acts automatically.

The fundamental difference between these notions is that the first is
an "instinctive" or "reflex"-type model and the latter is a "motivational" model. An instinctive theory sees sleep as a system like "nest
building" or "migration" or "mothering" of the young offspring. It
occurs because the appropriate behavior is elicited relative to the
circumstances of the surround and the time. It is not due to some
"loss" or "deprivation." The restorative model, on the contrary, in a
"motivational" matrix, sees sleep as a response to some increasing
buildup of noxious states or as a deprivation condition requiring us to
sleep in order to restore the lost "sustenance."

In the first model one seeks "causes" of sleep in the environment,
while in the latter the causes lie within the organism.

Unfortunately, when it comes to deciding between rival theories
there is usually no good way to do so. Certainly it is true in this case.
Both are linked with time. Both are concerned with the major
dimensions of sleep. Both work "innately" in relationship to internal
cues and the developed physiology of the organism. Neither has been
developed to the level at which predictions can be tested for accuracy.

We can, at this stage, only express a preference. I turned to the
behavioral model originally because of a few substantial puzzles about
"restoration." First, "what" is being diminished and, in turn, "re-

stored" has been so elusive that it has not been specifiable. The notions of the buildup of "toxins" and their removal have gradually retreated into such speculative places as a recovery of certain nerve endings associated with learning. Second, the recovery rate must be assumed to be different relative to different sleep behavior rather than predictive of these differences. By this we mean that short sleepers (either between or within species) must be assumed to have faster recovery rates, since they are necessarily awake for a longer period of time each 24 hours. For example, the recovery rate of an elephant that is awake some 20-plus hours a day must be much faster than that of a gorilla that is awake about 10 hours per day, since the first sleeps for only 4 hours and the latter for 14 hours.

I prefer the adaptive model for three major reasons. The first is that, as a psychologist, I am more naturally inclined to try to understand the relationship between the environment, past and present, and the behavior at hand. Second, it helps me to predict sleep behavior. As I have read about the wide range of sleep behaviors in animals, the "fit" of sleep to aid its survival in the food gathering matrix is, so far, a good one. Third, and most important, it is a model that helps me, at least, to understand human sleep better. Let me expand on this point as a sort of summary of the path we have followed through this book.

Human sleep as an adaptive response

What we have said generally about sleep is that we sleep as we do because we have inherited a pattern of behavior. It is innate, unlearned, and self-sustaining. It is an understandable, "law-abiding" biological system, containing its own built-in rules, with which we have been endowed as part of our human heritage. It is a precious gift that we may accept with as much grace as we have within us.

This adaptive system of sleep seems to fit very well the body of facts that we have reviewed in this book. An inherent biological system has at least six characteristics:

1. It is unlearned.
2. It is developmental in nature.
3. It is species specific but with a typical range of individual differences within species.
4. It is "law-abiding."
5. It is self-perpetuating.
6. It is adaptive in relation to the organism's environment.

Consider what we have learned about sleep. We have seen that sleep "unfolds" in its own time and way as the child grows from infancy to maturity. These patterns are distinct and occur with remarkable similarity across a wide range of conditions and attitudes, generation after generation. Each species, within limits of individual differences, follows its unique but common pattern.

Sleep, indeed, shows law-abiding characteristics, and these laws function in a self-perpetuating and adaptive manner. Sleep is systematically affected by what is done to it as a system. If we stay awake for a long time, we become sleepy; if we shorten sleep, we affect the kind of sleep we will get; if we go to sleep at a different time from the usual, sleep will be disrupted; if we are under threat or intensive stimulation, we will hold off sleep; if we distort the sleep structure, it will respond compensatorily; sleep will be disrupted by pathologies.

The system is both sensitive and self-protective, has its own requirements and demands, but is remarkably adaptive to our needs. In spite of becoming sleepy we can stay awake when we extend our wakefulness. Though disrupted by displacements in time, it will be reorganized. While ignoring routine variations in our world, it remains sensitive to "meaningful" variations in that world, both preceding and during sleep. When impacted by our own impositions on its structure, it struggles to offset these effects. Each of the specific examples could be reviewed, but I hope that these selected few are sufficient enough to help us better understand the nature of sleep as an inherent, evolutionarily developed system of biological functioning.

Implications

The function of sleep has been described as fulfilling an adaptive role in behavioral control. In each species, sleep evolved as a system of "nonresponse" in protection against a dangerous or ineffective response. From this point of view sleep is an inherent, innate biological heritage of man. We sleep as we do because we were so built over countless periods of time.

Like all biological functions, sleep has its innate course of development, is lawfully sensitive to its treatment, and self-protective in its ways. At the same time it is remarkably adaptive, within limits, to man's life-style within his environment. When permitted and not pushed, it unfolds and proceeds to perform effectively its ordained patterns. When pushed by our real or presumed needs it yields and bends but remembers and reminds us of its nature.

This chapter began with a wise quotation from Samuel Johnson. He called sleep a "gentle tyrant." This seems most apt. To live on the best terms with a "gentle tyrant" one must learn the rules by which he governs. Being gentle, he permits us certain freedoms to manifest our individual variations and differences; being a tyrant, he will not permit us to live in total freedom, and abuses carry their ultimate consequences. Although we may deplore "benevolent dictators" in our politics, this one seems efficient, is unlikely to be overthrown, and can best be lived with in peace.

15

Questions and answers

This last chapter consists of a series of questions that I have found occurring with remarkable frequency and consistency during question periods after lectures, phoned in to "talk show" appearances about sleep, at cocktail parties, on airplanes, or on other occasions when my area of research is revealed as sleep.

I have put them in their usual question form although I have eliminated the tone of the question, which is one of pure curiosity, embarrassment or, for some unfathomed reason, downright hostility. These latter forms characteristically begin "Don't you . . . ."

The answers vary from reasonably confident and certain through speculative to evasive. For this set of questions, as you will see, the tilt is toward the speculative-evasive end of the continuum since many of the questions, while often intriguing or interesting, are remote from the central core of the understanding and control of sleep itself. They generally represent rarities or their relationship to sleep is more apparent than real.

Such apologies over with, your questions, please.

Is hypnosis a form of sleep?

The answer is a clear unequivocal no if one uses the now most generally accepted definition of sleep, the EEG reading. The actively hypnotized person does not show any sleep signs in his EEG. The hypnotized subject, if left alone or specifically instructed to do so, may go into natural sleep. However, when he does, he is then asleep and no longer hypnotized, since the hypnotizer has lost command of the person.

The confusions between the two have stemmed from some parallels in conscious experiences and behavior. In both hypnosis and sleep, responses to the environment are selective and at a low level. On awakening from sleep and emerging from hypnosis, individuals remember little of what has occurred. We have seen, in the case of sleeptalking, that on the "edges" of sleep the person may be more suggestible. Individuals can be instructed to have a "dream" in hypnosis and recall that "dream." However similar these parallels, they are only similar in appearance and differ sharply in many ways. For example, the selective attention in hypnosis is achieved under the instruction of the hypnotizer. The recall of the dream in sleep is dependent upon a brain state (REM) and not on instruction. Suggestibility in the two states differs more in kind than degree. "Dreams" from the two states are qualitatively different.

There is some evidence that hypnotic suggestions can "penetrate" into sleep. If the person is hypnotized and given an instruction such as "Scratch your nose when you hear the word 'itch,' " that word, spoken to the sleeping subject, results in a nose-scratching well beyond chance. Studies of this type may well lead us to a better understanding of our "monitoring" capacity within sleep.

Can we learn during sleep?

Probably a little but not very much.

Hope to do things the easy way springs eternal. Each year an unknown but considerable number of sleep-learning devices are sold. These are records or tapes fed into earphones or placed under one's pillow. They typically purport to teach foreign languages. There is an extensive Russian literature on the successful application of sleep learning. From one report, an entire village had its learning of English facilitated by playing English phrases all night long over the state radio! Somewhat better controlled experiments in Russia have made strong claims for "hypnopaedia" (sleep learning).

Well-controlled studies conducted in the United States since the late 1940s using the EEG and presenting material only during certain sleep have consistently found almost no effect on morning testing of material. Items recalled were almost always associated with a period of wakefulness or very light sleep within sleep.

A review of the Russian literature revealed that their procedures differed in three ways from the Western studies: learning was best in "suggestible" subjects; strong "sets," or "suggestions," of recall were used; and the subjects were given considerable presleep practice in learning material by auditory input.

Two recent carefully designed studies conducted in the United States used a high degree of suggestion with suggestible subjects. Paired associates (a Russian word stood for an English word) were presented during the various sleep stages. The results were remarkably similar. There was essentially no "free recall" of the pairs or a correct response to the "stem," or Russian word. However, the subjects were able to "recognize" correct pairings better than chance expectancy. (One study gave the first word and asked which one of the 6 words had been paired; the other selected the appropriate pairings out of 10 words. Both did about 15 percent better than chance.)

Can we learn during sleep? It appears that suggestible subjects who are given strong "sets" to recall may *recognize* a small amount of material presented during sleep. This does not encourage the practical use of sleep learning. The form of learning is limited and the amount small. It is estimated that the same amount of recall may be obtained from a very few minutes while awake.

Can sleep be induced?

Sleep can, of course, be induced—certainly by staying awake for a long period of time and less certainly by drugs. However, the thrust of this question is usually directed at the use of mechanical or routine procedures such as monotonous sounds, records of rain on tin roofs, muscular relaxation exercises, hypnosis, the more recent "biofeedback" systems, or even "Russian sleep machines." The answer is, again, probably somewhat but really not much.

Sleep inducers may theoretically facilitate or evoke sleep in a number of ways operating singly or in combination (usually the latter):

1. Direct action on the central nervous system, i.e., stimulating some "sleep center."

2. Masking or reducing incompatible "nonsleep" stimuli and behavior.

3. Increasing or amplifying sleep-compatible behaviors.

4. Suggestion.

5. Developing sleep habits.

Take the old simple standbys of counting or attending to the clicking of a clock, or the internal variant—counting sheep. It is possible that the rhythmic input may evoke a central nervous system sleep response. Certainly by concentrating on the particular stimulus one is less likely to attend to thoughts about the day or attend to sounds which provide "nonsleep" responses. Then, lying with one's eyes closed in a relaxed position may help to induce sleep. The simple belief that this will bring sleep is likely to be helpful. Finally, if this behavior is always and only associated with falling asleep, a sleep habit may be promoted.

Given all that, can sleep be induced? First, it appears unlikely that a central nervous system can be "tripped" or a "button pushed." Direct electrical stimulation of *some very particular areas of the brain with some restricted frequencies* can result in somnolence. However, stimulation outside of these areas and with different frequencies within these areas leads to no response or to arousal. In some rare instances, particularly with lower animals, there is evidence of extreme external stimulation or conflict evoking sleep. However, no studies of sensory stimulation (by means of visual or auditory cues, or vibrations, etc.) have demonstrated a certain and automatic onset of sleep, and the direct stimulation studies would support a contrary position.

The next most direct route to sleep would be amplifying aspects of the sleep pattern. These would include "biofeedback" systems, various forms of muscular relaxation, or other physiological changes evoked, for instance, by drinking warm milk or changing the temperature of the surround. Biofeedback systems involve "feeding back" information about some physiological state such as the alpha rhythm, the heart rate, breathing, or muscular tension level in order that a person can better achieve a particular signaled state. We may also try to achieve these states by instruction or training programs in progressive relaxation ("First relax the legs, now the arms . . ." or "Breathe more slowly . . ."). There is little doubt that physiologically arranging oneself to take the sleep position should be helpful in getting to sleep. Certainly automating or "learning" to get into these positions is likely to be useful. Most of the relaxation systems carry with them the three additional advantages of any system: distraction, suggestion, and habit formation. Any individual success with any of the amplification systems may be due to those factors rather than to any direct effects. A warm shower before bed may result in a peripheral vascular response (the blood system going into the outer parts of the system) which may be "mimicking" what happens at sleep onset. The sleep response is thus "teased" into a quicker occurrence; or the person may believe that it helps; or the person may find this useful in "disconnecting" from the day's activities; or the routine may facilitate all of these things.

The use of monotonous sounds as a sleep inducer has been systematically studied. We took a group of students and had them come into the laboratory in the morning after a good night's sleep. As such they were "artificial insomniacs," since sleep was difficult to achieve. We divided them into 4 groups: the first received complete silence; the second, a constant tone; the third, a repeated tone; and the fourth, a repeated tone plus counting. The repeated tone was on for 2 seconds and off for 2 seconds. To control for a "suggestion" effect all groups were told that "research had shown that X condition was useful in producing sleep" and that we were studying the brain waves under that condition. They were given a sleep opportunity period of 45 minutes for 5 successive mornings.

The differences between the groups were not statistically significant but the two repeated-tone groups did differ from the group experiencing the silence and that experiencing a continuous tone. Although the repeated tones "facilitated" sleep, they could hardly be said effectively to induce sleep. The latencies were still longer than 10 minutes. The matter of habituation was interesting. Just sleeping in the laboratory for 5 days had a stronger effect than the tone differences (latency dropped from 25 minutes to 17 minutes). However, it appears that the "new" procedure—a tone—tended originally to disrupt sleep but to facilitate sleep after it had become familiar.

These data indicate that the presence of some types of repeated and monotonous tones may have a small but measurable effect in facilitating sleep. The effect is probably mediated through the person focusing on an irrelevant, noninterfering stimulation which results in a decreased effect of sleep-distracting stimuli. However, there is some possibility that suggestion was still operative. It is certainly easier to believe that a particular tone rather than silence "has been scientifically proved" to be sleep-inducing.

We can only guess and be logical about the role of belief or suggestion in relation to sleep induction. Obviously if a person doesn't believe that he can go to sleep in a particular stimulus situation he will have difficulties in going to sleep. If a "presumed" sleep inducer annoys or frightens him, sleep probability will also be reduced. On the positive side we are without the obvious data. The highest form of belief or suggestion would be hypnosis.

The use of an actual hypnotizer for sleep problems would be of only theoretical interest (unless one were married to or living with such a skilled person). Even here usefulness would be dependent upon the suggestibility of the sleeper-to-be and the skill of the hypnotizer. The hypnotic state achieved might result in a longer or shorter than natural sleep latency. The same would hold true for a "hypnotic record" or self-hypnosis. In both of the latter procedures, undoubtedly the "distraction" element and the habit pattern would be adjunctively involved. Posthypnotic suggestion would seem to hold the highest hope. The person under hypnosis would be told, "When you count to ten you will fall asleep" or some similar suggestion. On going to bed the individual would then count to ten, with the "implanted" belief of sleep following thereafter. Unfortunately, I know of no systematic study of this procedure.

Sleep "habits" are probably useful. Certainly a regularity of bedtime is helpful. When we add to this regularity a going-to-sleep routine—combing one's hair, saying one's prayers, drinking hot milk, reading one chapter in a non-required, not especially attention-engaging book—as "signals" for sleep, we are probably increasing sleep tendencies. With repetitions of signals followed by sleep, these signs become tendencies to "do" sleep rather than "do" something else rather than sleep. We are "learning" that these "mean" sleep, and that magnificent system of "habits" is put to use in our service.

We would point up this matter of habits by its contrary. If going to bed is "associated" with reviewing the day or reading a book we will not put down until we finish, then that is what going to bed is likely to elicit—not going to sleep. Do those things before you try to go to sleep!

Can sleep be induced? Probably not, but it can certainly be helped along its way.

Are there two types of sleep people— "night owls and day larks"?

Most of us know of people who say that they are night owls. They can't get to sleep until the wee hours of the morning and can't function very well before high noon. Is this some kind of sleep type, an inverted or displaced biological rhythm? Probably not. It is more likely to be a maintained social pattern of behavior.

We noted in Chapter 5 when talking about shifts of sleep-onset time that when shift workers change from sleeping at night to sleeping during the day, sleep was temporarily disrupted; then this sleep begins to reorganize itself. After a week or so they are sleeping during the day in the same way that they had been sleeping at night. Our best evidence indicates that sleep may be placed at any point within the 24 hours and will take its natural form at that point if there is an adequate amount and if there is some regularity of placement.

What does this say about the night owl? It says that through a pattern of beliefs, experiences, or choices he has developed a pattern of going to sleep at 4:00 A.M. He is a poor performer during the day because he can't have gotten enough sleep by 8:00 A.M. and he still needs to keep sleeping. However, there is no biological reason that he should not begin sleep four hours earlier and thus function effectively four hours earlier.

A story told to me by a colleague in sleep research illustrates this matter very well. A new medical resident in his hospital came to him for his expert advice on the resident's sleep problem. "Sir," he said, "I'm a night owl and I am in real trouble. I got through medical school easily. I studied all night while others were sleeping and because the books taught me well, I could doze through the daily lectures. They loved me as an intern because I took all the night shifts. But now I'm a resident and they expect me in the clinic at eight A.M. and I can't do it." My friend said, "You must keep going to sleep at four A.M. New York time regardless of the circumstances. Correct? I have a simple suggestion. Keep this up but shift your residency to Hawaii. You will then begin going to bed at ten P.M. Hawaii time—four A.M. New York time—and your problem is solved. Another possibility is to simply start going to bed—whether you sleep or not—at eleven P.M. in New York. Give that a try first for a few weeks and come back and see me if it doesn't work." The young resident didn't come back, didn't go to Hawaii, and he completed his residency. We don't know whether he stopped being an "owl" but we suspect that he did.

Can you use sleep deprivation to "brainwash" people?

We first have to decide what we mean by "brainwashing." The term has usually been associated with changing the statements and presumably the beliefs of political prisoners to those of their captors. The most dramatic examples were seen in the "confessions" during the Russian political trials of the 1930s and those of American prisoners during the Korean war. We mean in these instances more than just a changing of one's mind—which we all do every day—but a restructuring of one's basic beliefs.

We can begin by saying that changing one's beliefs is an active process achieved by systematically bringing to bear psychological forces which "reinforce" or reward a different set of beliefs, and, often, by "punishing" or at least not rewarding the formerly held beliefs. The poet W. H. Auden stated this dramatically: "Of course Behaviorism works. Give me a powerful electric shock and complete control over an individual and I'll have him reciting the Athanasian creed in public in a month."

The process of effective change is likely to be more complicated than Auden anticipated, but the point is that it is an active one. We cannot expect that, by simply keeping a person awake for any period of time, his beliefs will be the opposite of those which he formerly held.

Is sleep loss useful as a procedure to achieve brainwashing? I would have to guess that it would be an effective adjunct. The situation that one would want to create would be a state of helplessness and dependency upon the conditioner, and hence a situation in which the conditioner can supply a badly needed "reward." It would be most useful if this condition were a continuous one. It would also be useful if the procedure didn't have to show visible "damage" to the person— such as the loss of fingers or the like.

In an oversimplified picture, a "brainwashing" using sleep loss would go something like this. Sleep deprivation would be introduced by making sleep difficult to obtain; the use of bright lights, continued surveillance and stimulation, enforced standing or walking, deprivation of a place to lie down, very cold or hot conditions, etc., would all be helpful here. The prisoner would recite and "associate" his present beliefs with this condition. As sleep loss progressed, obtaining sleep would be dependent upon his rejection or denial of his current beliefs and gradual acceptance of contrary beliefs.

The effective aspects of this procedure are that it can be maintained as long as desirable, it can be used selectively ("bad" treatment when the prisoner is "bad," and "good" treatment when the prisoner is "good"), and there is the continual threat of reinstatement. It is probably a more powerful "weapon" than starvation for several reasons. The effects are less "understandable" and more "pressing" than those resulting from food deprivation. A person may "will" himself not to think about food, and the reward may not be as immediate or sharp. It is also likely to be more effective than physical punishment since it is more continuous, can be withdrawn more simply, and probably evokes less psychological resentment: "That monster is hurting me and I hate him" versus "I wish he would let me go to sleep."

Certainly a fully effective procedure would use sophisticated conditioning techniques across a wide range. However, sleep deprivation would probably be a particularly useful tool.

Can a person be "brainwashed" with sleep loss? We must first believe that a person *can* be "brainwashed." It is not unreasonable to believe that ideas can be changed in varying degrees depending upon the individual, the strength of his original beliefs, and the rewards associated with the changed beliefs. Under such circumstances loss of sleep alone would not be expected to change beliefs; however, sleep loss may be used as a very efficient procedure in the process of change.

Is hibernation sleeping?

There have been a large number of studies of hibernation, as well as a large number of studies of sleep, but few have related the two behaviors. One of the reasons for this is that our infallible guideline, the EEG, is of dubious help here. In deep hibernation the EEG is markedly reduced in its output and may even be "silent."

Hibernation occurs in a limited set of mammals in the face of extreme cold and a reduced food supply. However, these external cues alone are seldom sufficient to induce hibernation. Rather, it is a seasonal rhythm preceded by developing fatty body deposits and, often, a stored food supply. In some animals—for example, the American ground squirrel—hibernation will take place at the usual season even if the animal is kept in an environment of constant temperature and lighting with an ample food supply.

The length and degree of hibernation varies widely. The dormouse will typically hibernate from September to April, whereas the hedgehog may not begin hibernation until the year's end and may hibernate for less than three months. Some species remain essentially torpid throughout the hibernation while others, such as the golden hamster, "awake" about every three days and eat.

In most hibernators there is a sharp drop in body temperature, metabolism, heart rate, and respiration. This drop in temperature is internally determined rather than being a matching of the external temperature. Again, there are wide variations. The dormouse rolls up in a light ball, is completely torpid, is cold to the touch, and is so rigid that he can be rolled. The bear is in a sense not a true hibernator, since his body temperature is generally maintained and he is arousable. However, his heart rate is sharply reduced from even his low sleeping level of 40 beats per minute to 10 beats per minute and occasionally less. Bats in hibernation may breathe 20 to 25 times per minute for several minutes and not breathe at all for up to 8 minutes. This is in comparison with their normal rate of about 200 breaths per minute while active and is considerably lower than their breathing rate when asleep.

Hibernation, then, is a seasonal "nonresponse" which results in a marked degree of energy conservation in the face of adverse conditions. The bodily changes are similar to but far more marked than those that occur during sleep. It is tempting, however, to draw parallels between its functional role in adaptation and that ascribed to sleep in the preceding chapter.

How long are dreams?

We know that reported dreams may be a mere wisp of a scene or be elaborate reports which, when taken down, may extend over pages of record. This question usually is really asking: "How long does a dream take in real time?" Are they like the reputed "lifetimes" that flash before the drowning man or do they take up the same amount of time they would if we were awake?

The concept of the dream occurring in a moment stems from a very famous dream reported by the French physician Maury, who studied dreams in the early 1800s (Chapter 13). He dreamed an elaborate dream of being taken to the guillotine during the French Revolution and being beheaded. He inferred that his dream and others occurred in the split second of awakening because he had been awakened by a bed rail falling on his neck. This fits well with the common experience of the awakening stimulus being a logical part of the dream: the alarm clock signal being the end of a class we were dreaming about, the bark of a dog being a part of an elaborate outdoor jaunt.

We will perhaps never know with certainty the answers to these questions. Every evidence points to the presence of dream scenes throughout the REM periods and not as simply awakening phenomena. The inclusion of the awakening stimulus into the dream seems to be merely a continuation of the "free associative" character of dream content. If Maury's bed rail had not fallen, he might never have been beheaded but he might have "turned into" the executioner. As for the time span of the dream, I believe that the dream "time" is analogous to time in imagination. We can imagine a shipboard trip to England—embarking, the cabin, the promenade, the bar, the steward, the dinner, the trunks, the customs—in one great rush of feeling. I can also extend any element of that passage across long intervals of real time—one evening of dinner, the wines, the dancing, the weather, the individuals of that evening. How long, then, is my shipboard "dream"? A second or an hour are equally plausible answers.

Where can I learn more about sleep?

The problems in answering this question are several and different in kind. As one becomes more deeply involved in a particular topic the literature quickly becomes very technical and the recent findings widely scattered in a range of journals that are not readily accessible (in 1973 articles on sleep appeared in 164 different journals). Broader and more summarizing books are often dated soon after publication by the rapid changes in the field.

Readers with broader interests may wish to read the "Old Testament" of sleep research—Nathaniel Kleitman's *Sleep and Wakefulness* (2nd. ed., University of Chicago Press, 1963). This is a scholarly and encyclopedic summary of all the relevant research in sleep through 1963 and contains 4,337 references. *Sleep and Dreams* by Gay Luce and Jules Segal (Coward-McCann, 1966) was written for a general reading audience. This well-written book summarizes the active field of sleep research and its ongoing findings in the mid-1960s. A very recent book by Dr. Ernest Hartmann published in paperback by Yale University Press (*The Functions of Sleep*, 1974) combines interesting data drawn from animal studies, clinical studies, and biochemical studies about the functions of sleep. It is described as (and is) "written clearly enough for the layman to understand [and] is nonetheless a sophisticated theoretical contribution to the literature on sleep."

On specialized topics discussed in this book but, again, written for the general reading public three books should be considered. Luce and Segal have also written an exciting book on *Insomnia* (Coward-McCann, 1968). There have been two recent books on dreams. One by Ann Faraday, entitled *Dream Power* (Coward, McCann & Geoghegan, 1972) is specifically concerned with dream interpretation and is written by a clinical psychologist who began her work with laboratory analyses of dreams. It has sold more than 500,000 copies. An anthology about dreams has been recently published. The *New World of Dreams* (Macmillan, 1974) edited by Woods and Greenhouse, includes articles ranging from excerpts of ancient Egyptian papyri to the most recent REM sleep studies.

I would direct the reader who wishes to pursue some particular topic in technical detail, as I would any serious student, to the library. Beyond the card catalogue, which may yield a number of the more than two dozen books on sleep and dreams published in the last decade, I would commend recent copies of *Psychological Abstracts*. This publication of the American Psychological Association abstracts all of the articles of interest to psychologists. Under the topic "Sleep and Dreams" one will find more than 1,000 articles abstracted and indexed for the year 1974. These articles range from analytical interpretation of dreams to urinary excretions during sleep.

Index

A

Adaptiveness, 58, 158–59, 162–64
Alcohol, 94
Alpha rhythm, 12, 14
Animals, 15, 152, 159–60
Age:
  infancy, 29–32
  noise and, 57–58
  old age, 35–36, 82
  pre-school, 32–34, 73
  young adult, 19–23

B

Bed wetting, 77–78
Brain washing, 172–73
Brain waves, 11

C

Cardiovascular problems, 84
Clinics, 105–7

D

Daytime activities, (*see* Pre-sleep
  conditions)
Deprivation:
  total, 119–27
  partial, 129–32
  REM (*see* REM sleep)
Depth, 12, 57
Dreams:
  descriptions, 137–42
  dream work, 147
  interpretation, 146–49
  length, 175–76
  omens, 144–45
  viewpoints, 143–50
  REM, 150–54
Drugs, 90–98, 112–14

E

EEG (electroencephalogram),
  11–14, 15–16
Encephalitis lethargica, 81